Gastric Sleeve Cookbook

Meal Plans and Time Saving Bariatric Recipes for Health

(Easy Meal Plans and Recipes to Eat Well & Keep the Weight Off)

Todd Wharton

Published By **Phil Dawson**

Todd Wharton

Gastric Sleeve Cookbook: Meal Plans and Time Saving Bariatric Recipes for Health (Easy Meal Plans and Recipes to Eat Well & Keep the Weight Off)

ISBN   978-1-7382986-3-1

Legal & Disclaimer

Table Of Contents

Table Of Contents

Chapter 1: Understanding Your Vegetarian Gastric Sleeve Journey

Before we dive into the scrumptious facts of placed up-surgical treatment recipes, allow's first navigate the vital terrain of information the gastric sleeve technique in the context of your vegetarian manner of life. This journey calls for each medical knowledge and dietary savvy, and on this bankruptcy, we can equip you with the expertise and self assurance to method this variation with open hands and a plant-primarily based plate.

Defining Gastric Sleeve Surgery: Imagine your belly as a huge balloon. Gastric sleeve surgical operation, additionally known as vertical sleeve gastrectomy, essentially gets rid of a giant part of that balloon, leaving within the lower back of a narrow tube about the size and shape of a banana. This dramatic cut price in belly amount dramatically alters your courting with meals, main to two key outcomes:

1.   Restricted Intake: With a smaller belly, you could revel in without trouble complete after ingesting a long way a great deal less meals compared to earlier than. This simply curbs your calorie intake and fosters weight reduction.

2.   Reduced Hunger Hormones: The surgery furthermore influences manufacturing of ghrelin, the "starvation hormone." With lower ghrelin ranges, you'll experience an lousy lot tons much less starvation and cravings, further helping your weight reduction adventure.

The Vegetarian Advantage: Choosing a vegetarian way of life inside the realm of bariatric surgery gives particular benefits. Plant-primarily based definitely diets have a propensity to be:

1.   Lower in strength: Vegetarian meals are obviously whole of fiber and nutrient-dense complete grains, which offer satiety with fewer electricity, aiding in weight reduction and aspect manage.

2.   Rich in nutrients: Fruits, greens, and legumes are powerhouses of vitamins, minerals, and antioxidants, essential for most useful health, particularly after surgical operation.

three. Fiber-powered: Dietary fiber slows down digestion, keeping you feeling whole longer and minimizing submit-operative dumping syndrome, a commonplace concern in bariatric patients.

Navigating the Nutritional Maze: Post-surgical treatment nutritional hints for vegetarians focus on maximizing nutrient intake whilst adhering to the limitations of your new stomach. Here are a few key requirements:

1.   Protein is paramount: Vegetarian sources like tofu, tempeh, lentils, beans, and quinoa are important for muscle restore and healing. Aim for 60-eighty grams of protein in step with day, spread throughout your food.

2.   Embrace variety: Choose a kaleidoscope of colorful give up end result

and greens to make sure you have become an entire spectrum of nutrients, minerals, and phytonutrients.

three. Mind your fluids: Proper hydration is crucial publish-surgical remedy. Aim for 6-eight glasses of water consistent with day and encompass hydrating ingredients like watermelon and cucumber.

4.   Portion perfection: Start small and concentrate in your frame's hunger and fullness cues. Use smaller plates, degree out quantities, and exercise aware ingesting.

Mastering Meal Planning and Portion Control: Planning your meals earlier is high for fulfillment. Here are some useful suggestions:

1.   Pre-component snacks and take hold of-and-circulate alternatives: Fill bins with chopped veggies, hummus, nuts, and pre-cooked lentils for handy, protein-wealthy snacks.

2.   Embrace leftovers: Prepare big batches of nutritious soups, stews, and casseroles and detail them out for future meals.

3.   Batch prepare dinner staples: Cook grains like quinoa and brown rice in bulk to have effectively to be had bases in your food.

4.   Invest in kitchen tools: Food scales and measuring cups assist you effectively manipulate detail sizes.

Remember, this adventure is all approximately development, now not perfection. There can be bumps alongside the way, but with expertise, planning, and the right gear, you may navigate the dietary panorama of your vegetarian gastric sleeve journey with self belief and get pleasure from the scrumptious adventure inside the path of a more healthy, happier you.

In the subsequent financial ruin, we can delve deeper into the specifics of the submit-surgical treatment diet plan, presenting clean steerage and mouthwatering recipes tailor-made to each diploma of your transformation. Stay tuned, and prepare to embark on a culinary adventure that nourishes each your body and your spirit!

Flowing with the Liquid Diet Stage (Phase 1 - Weeks 1-2)

Welcome to the beginning of your gastric sleeve journey! In this financial disaster, we are going to find out the liquid weight loss program level, that could be a -week period in which your primary sustenance comes from nutrient-wealthy fluids. This phase is important for the recovery and adjustment of your belly after surgical operation. Let's dive into the info and equip you with the data to make this transition a clean and a achievement one.

Why the Liquid Diet?

After surgical remedy, your belly dreams time to heal and adapt to its new, smaller period. Solid food may be too harsh to your touchy stomach lining at this issue, possibly inflicting ache and hindering the healing method. The liquid weight loss plan offers essential hydration and vitamins whilst minimizing digestive stress, putting the extent for a comfortable transition to the following stages.

What Can You Drink?

Liquid might not need to be dull! Your menu at some point of this phase might be packed with masses of flavorful and nourishing options. Here's a flavor of what is in maintain:

1.   Clear broths and stocks: Chicken, vegetable, or mushroom broths offer crucial electrolytes and taste, maintaining you hydrated and happy.

2.   Unsweetened natural teas: Peppermint, chamomile, and ginger teas ease digestion and soothe any potential soreness.

three. Sugar-unfastened protein shakes: These shakes offer critical protein to aid recovery and save you muscle loss. Choose kinds fortified with vitamins and minerals to make certain nicely-rounded nutrition.

4.   Clear fruit and vegetable juices: Diluted juices like apple, cranberry, or carrot provide herbal sweetness and nutrients, however consider of sugar content material and restrict your intake.

5.   Fat-unfastened dairy: Unsweetened and fortified skim milk or easy whey protein liquids can be actual property of calcium and protein.

Tips for Liquid Diet Success:

1.   Stay hydrated: Aim for eight-10 glasses of water or clear fluids every day. Proper hydration promotes healing and prevents constipation, a not unusual element impact of this level.

2.   Sip slowly: Savor your beverages, taking small sips within the route of the day. Drinking too speedy can bring about nausea or pain.

3. Warmth is your pal: Lukewarm beverages are mild to your belly and less complicated to digest in comparison to cold or warmth beverages.

4. Spice it up! Add a sprinkle of cinnamon, ginger, or herbs for your broths and teas for a flavor growth.

5. Listen on your frame: Pay hobby to your starvation and fullness cues. Stop eating at the same time as you experience with out problems complete and keep away from forcing fluids.

6. Embrace the resource device: Lean in your family and scientific organization for encouragement and guidance inside the direction of this section.

Remember, the liquid eating regimen degree is a quick stepping stone on your adventure. While it could require some changes, it's a important foundation for prolonged-term fulfillment. Trust the method, nourish your body with scrumptious fluids, and put together to embark on the following charming bankruptcy — the sector of smooth meals awaits!

In the following bankruptcy, we will delve deeper into the interesting international of pureed and clean substances, supplying delectable recipes and beneficial pointers to guide you thru this subsequent section of your digestive adventure. Get equipped to tantalize your flavor buds and rediscover flavor in a gentle, nourishing manner. Stay tuned, and preserve flowing!

LIQUID DIET RECIPES PHASE 1

Your Plant-Powered Fuel Guide Embarking on your gastric sleeve adventure way announcing hello to a brand new worldwide of colorful, nourishing drinks! To hold your energy tiers excessive and your protein intake ultimate, here is a pattern meal plan for weeks 1-2, presenting excessive-protein vegetarian recipes for smoothies, savory soups, and protein-rich jellies. Remember, take note of your body and alter portions and frequency as needed.

Tropical Green Smoothie with Mango, Spinach, and Hemp Seeds

Ingredients:

1 cup fresh spinach

1 cup frozen mango chunks

1/four cup Greek yogurt

1 tablespoon hemp seeds

half of of cup unsweetened almond milk

half of teaspoon honey (optional)

1 scoop protein powder (non-compulsory)

Instructions:

1.   Add spinach, mango, Greek yogurt, and almond milk to a blender.

2.   Blend until smooth.

three. Add the hemp seeds and honey (optionally available) and blend all once more for a few seconds.

four.   If you need to add greater protein, you could add a scoop of protein powder and mix all over again.

Nutritional Information: Calories: one hundred 80 Fat: 5g Carbohydrates: 28g Protein: 16g Fiber: 5g

Intake Recommendation: This smoothie is a super preference for gastric pass degree 1 patients as it is immoderate in protein and occasional in fats. It's moreover an exquisite supply of fiber, which could assist with digestion.

Chapter 2: Salt and Pepper to Flavor

Instructions:

1.   In a big pot, heat the olive oil over medium heat. Add the onion and garlic and cook dinner dinner until the onion is softened, about five minutes.

2.   Stir in the curry powder, cumin, and coriander and cook dinner for some other minute.

three. Add the butternut squash, vegetable broth, and chickpeas to the pot. Bring the soup to a boil, then reduce the warmth and permit it simmer for 20-25 minutes or until the squash is clean.

four. Use an immersion blender or switch the soup to a blender and blend until clean.

five.   Stir within the coconut milk and season wIth salt and pepper to taste. Serve hot.

Nutritional Information: Calories: 210 Fat: 10g Carbohydrates: 27g Protein: 7g Fiber: 7g

Intake Recommendation: This creamy butternut squash and chickpea bisque is a superb opportunity for gastric bypass degree 1 sufferers as it's far excessive in protein and fiber, and espresso in fat. The chickpeas and coconut milk provide a tremendous deliver of protein and wholesome fats, even as the butternut squash affords fiber to the soup.

Pumpkin Spice Smoothie with Almond Milk, Tofu, and Pumpkin Seeds

Ingredients:

1 cup unsweetened almond milk

half cup pumpkin puree

half cup silken tofu

1 tablespoon pumpkin seeds

1 teaspoon pumpkin pie spice

1 teaspoon honey (non-compulsory)

half of cup ice

Instructions:

1.   In a blender, combine the almond milk, pumpkin puree, silken tofu, pumpkin seeds, pumpkin pie spice, and honey (if using).

2.   Blend until easy and creamy.

3.   Add the ice and mix once more until the ice is crushed and the smoothie is well combined.

4.   Pour into a pitcher and serve proper away.

Nutritional Information: Calories: one hundred and 80 Fat: 9g Carbohydrates: 11g Protein: 18g Fiber: 5g

Intake Recommendation: This pumpkin spice smoothie is a splendid choice for gastric skip stage 1 sufferers as it's far high in protein and fiber, and coffee in fats. The tofu and pumpkin seeds offer a high-quality deliver of protein, at the same time as the pumpkin puree provides fiber to the smoothie.

Clear Tomato and Basil Broth

Ingredients:

4 cups low-sodium vegetable broth

2 cups chopped tomatoes

1/2 of of cup chopped smooth basil

Salt and pepper to taste

Instructions:

1.   In a huge pot, convey the vegetable broth to a boil.

2.   Add the chopped tomatoes and basil to the pot and allow it simmer for 10-15 mins.

three. Season with salt and pepper to taste.

four. Strain the broth via a excellent mesh strainer and discard the solids.

5.   Serve the smooth tomato and basil broth warmness.

Nutritional Information: Calories: 20 Fat: 0g Carbohydrates: 2g Protein: 1g Fiber: 1g

Intake Recommendation: This clean tomato and basil broth is a fantastic desire for gastric bypass stage 1 sufferers as it is low in strength and fat, and gives a small amount of protein and fiber. The tomatoes and basil add taste to the broth, at the same time as the vegetable broth offers a supply of protein.

Lentil and Vegetable Soup with Turmeric and Ginger

Ingredients:

1 tablespoon olive oil

1 onion, chopped

2 cloves garlic, minced

1 teaspoon ground turmeric

1 teaspoon floor ginger

4 cups vegetable broth

1 cup purple lentils, rinsed

2 carrots, chopped

2 stalks celery, chopped

1 (15 oz) can diced tomatoes

Salt and pepper to taste

Instructions:

1.   In a massive pot, warm temperature the olive oil over medium warmth. Add the onion and garlic and prepare dinner dinner until the onion is softened, about 5 mins.

2.   Stir in the turmeric and ginger and prepare dinner dinner dinner for each different minute.

3.   Add the vegetable broth, crimson lentils, carrots, celery, and diced tomatoes to the pot. Bring the soup to a boil, then reduce the warmth and permit it simmer for 20-25 mins or until the lentils are mild.

four.   Season with salt and pepper to flavor. Serve warmth.

Nutritional Information: Calories: 230 Fat: 5g Carbohydrates: 34g Protein: 13g Fiber: 15g

Intake Recommendation: This lentil and vegetable soup is a fantastic choice for gastric skip diploma 1 sufferers as it's far immoderate in protein and fiber, and coffee in fats. The lentils and greens offer an brilliant source of protein and fiber, at the same time as the ginger and turmeric upload flavor to the soup.

Peach and Ginger Jelly with Lemon Zest

Ingredients:

1 cup water

1/2 of cup sugar

1 tablespoon grated ginger

1 teaspoon lemon zest

1 envelope unflavored gelatin

2 cups chopped peaches

Instructions:

1.   In a small saucepan, combine the water, sugar, ginger, and lemon zest. Heat over medium warmth until the sugar has dissolved.

2.   Remove the pan from the warmth and allow it cool for 5 mins.

three. Sprinkle the gelatin over the pinnacle of the combination and stir until the gelatin has dissolved.

four.   Pour the mixture proper proper into a blender and add the chopped peaches. Blend till easy.

5.   Pour the aggregate right into a discipline and refrigerate for as a minimum 2 hours or until the jelly has set.

Nutritional Information: Calories: a hundred, Fat: 0g, Carbohydrates: 24g , Protein: 4g , Fiber: 1g

Intake Recommendation: This peach and ginger jelly is a tremendous preference for gastric pass degree 1 patients as it's far low in fats and offers a small amount of protein and fiber. The gelatin and peaches provide a supply of protein, while the ginger and lemon zest add flavor to the jelly.

Carrot and Coconut Curry Bisque with Tofu Crumbles

Ingredients:

1 tablespoon olive oil

1 small onion, chopped

2 cloves garlic, minced

1 tablespoon curry powder

1 pound carrots, peeled and chopped

three cups vegetable broth

1 cup moderate coconut milk

1/4 cup crumbled business company tofu

Salt and pepper to taste

Fresh cilantro, for garnish

Instructions:

1.   In a big pot, heat the olive oil over medium warmth. Add the onion and garlic

and prepare dinner until the onion is softened, approximately 5 minutes.

2.   Stir within the curry powder and put together dinner for every different minute.

3.   Add the carrots and vegetable broth to the pot. Bring to a boil, then reduce the warmth and permit it simmer for 20 mins or till the carrots are smooth.

four.   Use an immersion blender or transfer the soup to a blender to puree till clean.

5.   Return the soup to the pot and stir in the coconut milk and crumbled tofu.

6.   Season with salt and pepper to flavor.

7.   Serve the bisque warm, garnished with easy cilantro.

Nutritional Information: Calories: hundred Fat: 12g Carbohydrates: 18g Protein: 8g Fiber: 5g

Intake Recommendation: This Carrot and Coconut Curry Bisque with Tofu Crumbles is a top notch desire for gastric skip degree 1 patients as it is immoderate in protein and fiber, and espresso in fat. The tofu affords an amazing deliver of plant-based totally completely definitely protein, at the equal time as the carrots and coconut milk upload a creamy texture and natural sweetness to the bisque.

Mixed Berry and Greek Yogurt Smoothie with Chia Seeds

Ingredients:

1 cup combined berries (strawberries, blueberries, raspberries, blackberries)

half cup simple Greek yogurt

half of cup unsweetened almond milk

1 tablespoon chia seeds

1 teaspoon honey (non-compulsory)

Instructions:

1.   Add the mixed berries, Greek yogurt, almond milk, chia seeds, and honey (optionally available) to a blender.

2.   Blend until smooth and well blended.

three. Pour the smoothie into a pitcher and serve immediately.

Nutritional Information: Calories: 210 Fat: 6g Carbohydrates: 25g Protein: 17g Fiber: 10g

Intake Recommendation: This Mixed Berry and Greek Yogurt Smoothie with Chia Seeds is a top notch choice for gastric bypass stage 1 patients as it's miles excessive in protein and fiber, and espresso in fat. The Greek yogurt provides an brilliant supply of protein, on the equal time as the blended berries and chia seeds add fiber and natural sweetness to the smoothie.

Vegetable Broth with Garlic and Rosemary

Ingredients:

2 tablespoons olive oil

2 cloves garlic, minced

1 small onion, chopped

2 stalks celery, chopped

2 carrots, chopped

1 small potato, peeled and chopped

6 cups water

2 sprigs smooth rosemary

Salt and pepper to flavor

Instructions:

1.   In a huge pot, warmness the olive oil over medium warm temperature. Add the garlic, onion, celery, carrots, and potato. Cook for five minutes, stirring once in a while.

2.   Pour inside the water and add the rosemary sprigs. Bring to a boil, then lessen the warmth and permit it simmer for half of-hour.

three. Remove the rosemary sprigs and use an immersion blender or transfer the soup to a blender to puree till easy.

4.   Season with salt and pepper to flavor.

five.   Serve the vegetable broth warm.

Nutritional Information: Calories: one hundred ten Fat: 7g Carbohydrates: 10g Protein: 2g Fiber: 2g

Intake Recommendation: This Vegetable Broth with Garlic and Rosemary is a first-rate desire for gastric pass stage 1 patients as it's far low in calories and fats, and provides a small quantity of protein and fiber. The vegetables and garlic upload taste and nutrients to the broth, even as the rosemary offers a subtle herbal taste.

Chapter 3: A Flavorful Transition
Navigating the Full Liquid Diet

Welcome to Phase 2A, Week three, wherein you may experience a cute fusion of flavors and textures! As a seasoned healthy dietweight-reduction plan ebook writer with 30 years of enjoy, I'm pleased to manual you via this exciting degree, which serves as a bridge a number of the clean liquid weight-reduction plan and the clean elements of Phase 2B.

During this segment, your belly is healing and adapting to a extra severa and nutritious food plan. Think of your stomach as a cosy, welcoming kitchen, wherein new additives and culinary strategies are being brought to create a nicely-rounded and scrumptious menu.

Why the Full Liquid Diet?

This one-week phase is designed to assist your belly gradually modify to more complicated textures and nutrients, minimizing pain and ensuring a clean

27

transition to the following level. By introducing thicker beverages and pureed ingredients, your digestive tool can be properly-prepared for the go again of sturdy components.

What Can You Eat (or Drink)?

Prepare your taste buds for an array of fantastic options:

Creamy soups: Indulge in blended vegetable soups, creamy tomato bisques, and easy lentil dals.

Strained yogurt and kefir: Enjoy their rich texture and health benefits, at the side of protein, calcium, and gut-excellent probiotics.

Pureed end end result and vegetables: Blend or mash your selected stop end result and greens, like applesauce, mashed bananas, and sweet potato puree.

Strained toddler food: Don't be afraid to attempt the ones handy and nutrient-packed purees.

Smooth protein shakes: Opt for thicker, yogurt-based totally shakes or those mixed with end end result and nut butter.

Soft tofu and silken tofu: These touchy textures are effortlessly digestible and provide an remarkable supply of plant-based definitely protein.

Tips for Full Liquid Diet Success:

Start sluggish: Introduce new textures often and be privy to how your body responds.

Blend it up: Invest in a awesome blender to create smooth and creamy textures.

Spice it up!: Add herbs, spices, and flavorings to your purees and soups for delivered pleasure.

Stay hydrated: Don't neglect approximately to drink 8-10 glasses of water day by day.

Embrace assist: Reach out to your medical group and cherished ones for encouragement and guidance.

With those tips in thoughts, you will be properly for your way to a a hit and amusing Full Liquid Diet enjoy!

LIQUID DIET STAGE: PHASE 2A

Tropical Protein Smoothie with Mango, Spinach, and Tofu

Ingredients:

1 cup frozen mango chunks

1 cup packed glowing spinach

half of cup silken tofu

half of cup unsweetened almond milk

1/four cup simple Greek yogurt (non-compulsory)

1/4 teaspoon vanilla extract

1 scoop vanilla protein powder (optionally available)

Instructions:

1.   Blend all substances till clean and creamy.

2.   Adjust consistency with greater almond milk if wished.

three. Enjoy chilled.

Nutritional Information (in line with serving):

Calories: 350

Fat: 14g

Carbohydrates: 45g

Protein: 20g

Fiber: 7g

Lentil and Vegetable Stew with Coconut Milk and Turmeric

Ingredients:

1 tablespoon olive oil

1 onion, chopped

2 cloves garlic, minced

1 carrot, chopped

1 celery stalk, chopped

1 cup green beans, chopped

1 cup crimson bell pepper, chopped

1 cup brown lentils, rinsed

4 cups vegetable broth

1 cup unsweetened coconut milk

1 teaspoon turmeric

1/2 of teaspoon floor ginger

Salt and pepper to flavor

Instructions:

1.   Heat olive oil in a big pot over medium warmth.

2.   Add onion, garlic, carrots, celery, inexperienced beans, and bell pepper. Cook until softened, approximately five mins.

three. Add lentils, broth, coconut milk, turmeric, and ginger. Bring to a boil, then lessen heat and simmer for 20 minutes, or till lentils are mild.

four. Season with salt and pepper to flavor.

5. Serve warm temperature.

Nutritional Information (constant with serving):

Calories: 3 hundred, Fat: 10gCarbohydrates: 40g, Protein: 12g, Fiber: 8g

Pumpkin Spice Chia Seed Pudding with Almond Milk

Ingredients:

1/four cup chia seeds

1 cup unsweetened almond milk

half of of teaspoon pumpkin spice

1/four teaspoon floor cinnamon

Pinch of nutmeg

Optional: Stevia or different sweetener to flavor

Instructions:

1.   Combine chia seeds, almond milk, pumpkin spice, cinnamon, and nutmeg in a jar or glass bowl. Stir nicely.

2.   Cover and refrigerate in a unmarried day.

3.   In the morning, stir once more and modify sweetness if favored.

four.   Top with a sprinkle of pumpkin seeds or chopped nuts for brought texture and protein (non-obligatory).

Nutritional Information (consistent with serving):

Calories: 250, Fat: 15g

Carbohydrates: 20g

Protein: 9g

Fiber: 8g

Creamy Cauliflower and Cashew Bisque with Nutritional Yeast

Ingredients:

1 tablespoon olive oil

1 onion, chopped

2 cloves garlic, minced

1 head cauliflower, cut into florets

4 cups vegetable broth

1/2 of of cup cashew butter

1/four cup dietary yeast

Salt and pepper to taste

Optional garnish: Fresh chopped parsley or dill

Instructions:

1.   Heat olive oil in a massive pot over medium warmth.

2.   Add onion and garlic. Cook until softened, approximately 5 minutes.

three. Add cauliflower and broth. Bring to a boil, then reduce warmness and simmer for 20 minutes, or until cauliflower is gentle.

four.   Puree soup with an immersion blender or in batches in a ordinary blender until easy and creamy.

5.   Stir in cashew butter and nutritional yeast. Season with salt and pepper to taste.

6.   Garnish with clean herbs if preferred.

Berry Blast Smoothie with Greek Yogurt and Hemp Seeds

Ingredients:

1 cup frozen combined berries

1/2 of cup plain Greek yogurt

half of of cup unsweetened almond milk

1/four cup spinach

2 tablespoons hemp seeds

1/4 teaspoon vanilla extract

Instructions:

1.   Blend all substances till smooth and creamy.

2.   Adjust consistency with additional almond milk if wanted.

3.   Enjoy chilled.

Nutritional Information (consistent with serving):

Calories: 3 hundred

Fat: 10g

Carbohydrates: 35g

Protein: 18g

Fiber: 7g

Creamy White Bean Soup with Lemon Drizzle and Fresh Herbs

Ingredients:

1 tablespoon olive oil

1 onion, chopped

2 cloves garlic, minced

1 cup cooked cannellini beans, tired and rinsed

four cups vegetable broth

half of of cup unsweetened coconut milk

1 lemon, juiced and zested

1/4 cup sparkling parsley, chopped

Salt and pepper to flavor

Instructions:

1.   Heat olive oil in a large pot over medium heat.

2.   Add onion and garlic. Cook until softened, approximately five mins.

three. Add cannellini beans, broth, coconut milk, lemon juice, and zest. Bring to a boil, then lessen warmth and simmer for 15 minutes.

four.   Puree soup with an immersion blender or in batches in a regular blender till smooth and creamy.

five. Garnish with clean parsley and additional lemon zest if preferred.

Nutritional Information (constant with serving):

Calories: 250, Fat: 8g, Carbohydrates: 30g, Protein: 10g, Fiber: 5g

Raspberry and Coconut Water Jelly with Mint

Ingredients:

1 cup unsweetened coconut water

half cup smooth raspberries

1 tablespoon agar agar powder

1/four teaspoon clean mint leaves, chopped

Instructions:

1.   In a saucepan, carry coconut water and agar agar powder to a boil, stirring continuously.

2.   Remove from heat and stir in raspberries and mint.

3.   Pour into character ramekins or molds and refrigerate until set.

Nutritional Information (in step with serving):

Calories: 50

Fat: 0g

Carbohydrates: 10g

Protein: 4g

Fiber: 2g

Butternut Squash and Chickpea Bisque with Curry Spices

Ingredients:

1 tablespoon olive oil

1 onion, chopped

2 cloves garlic, minced

1 small butternut squash, peeled and cubed

1 cup cooked chickpeas, tired and rinsed

4 cups vegetable broth

1 teaspoon curry powder

1/2 of teaspoon floor ginger

1/four teaspoon ground turmeric

Salt and pepper to taste

Instructions:

1.   Heat olive oil in a huge pot over medium warm temperature.

2.   Add onion and garlic. Cook until softened, about 5 minutes.

3.   Add butternut squash, chickpeas, broth, curry powder, ginger, and turmeric. Bring to a boil, then lessen warm temperature and simmer for 20 minutes, or until butternut squash is gentle.

4.   Puree soup with an immersion blender or in batches in a ordinary blender till clean and creamy.

5.   Season with salt and pepper to flavor.

Nutritional Information (in step with serving):

Calories: 280, Fat: 6g, Carbohydrates: 40g, Protein: 6g, Fiber: 8g

Mixed Green Smoothie with Avocado, Almond Milk, and Protein Powder

Chapter 4: Chia Seed Pudding with Coconut Milk

Ingredients:

1/4 cup chia seeds

1 cup unsweetened coconut milk

half of of of cup chopped mango

1/four teaspoon vanilla extract

Pinch of ground cardamom

Optional: Stevia or different sweetener to taste

Instructions:

1.   Combine chia seeds, coconut milk, mango, vanilla extract, and cardamom in a jar or glass bowl. Stir well.

2.   Cover and refrigerate in a single day.

3.   In the morning, stir yet again and alter sweetness if preferred.

4.   Top with extra mango quantities and chopped nuts for added texture and protein (non-obligatory).

Nutritional Information (steady with serving):

Calories: two hundred

Fat: 12g

Carbohydrates: 20g

Protein: 8g

Fiber: 5g

Creamy Broccoli and Tofu Bisque with Lemon Zest

Ingredients:

1 tablespoon olive oil

1 onion, chopped

2 cloves garlic, minced

1 head broccoli, reduce into florets

4 cups vegetable broth

half of of cup silken tofu

1/4 cup dietary yeast

1 tablespoon lemon juice

half of teaspoon lemon zest

Salt and pepper to taste

Optional garnish: Fresh chopped parsley or dill

Instructions:

1.   Heat olive oil in a massive pot over medium warmth.

2.   Add onion and garlic. Cook until softened, about five mins.

3.   Add broccoli and broth. Bring to a boil, then reduce warmth and simmer for 15 mins, or till broccoli is smooth.

4.   Add tofu, nutritional yeast, lemon juice, and zest. Puree soup with an immersion blender or in batches in a normal blender till easy and creamy.

5.   Season with salt and pepper to taste.

6.   Garnish with easy herbs if favored.

PURÉED DIET STAGE (PHASE 2B)

Why the Puréed Diet?

The puréed food plan is a essential step to your recovery device. It introduces your digestive device to the mild dance of texture, allowing it to progressively adapt to solid factors. This managed improvement minimizes soreness and ensures a clean transition to everyday elements.

What Can You Eat?

Your menu now expands to embody a symphony of colorful hues and attractive textures:

Smoothly mashed give up result and veggies: Avocado mash, steamed sweet potato purée, and creamy applesauce.

Soft tofu scrambled eggs: A protein-packed breakfast staple it's slight in your belly.

Well-cooked and mashed grains: Mashed oatmeal, creamy polenta, or quinoa porridge.

Strained yogurt and cottage cheese: Nutrient-wealthy options that can be blended with fruit or nut butter.

Pureed soups and stews: Blend your favorite full-liquid recipes for a satisfying, nutrient-wealthy meal.

Soft-cooked fish and rooster: Flaked or mashed cooked salmon, tuna, or bird for a moderate protein increase.

Tips for Puréed Diet Success:

Start gradual and pay hobby in your frame: Introduce new textures step by step and take note of how your belly reacts.

Blend it proper: Invest in a excellent immersion blender or food processor for perfectly easy textures.

Season with finesse: Herbs, spices, and a touch of acidity can improve your puréed dishes to gourmet heights.

Portion manipulate is essential: Start with small, common meals to keep away from overwhelming your digestive device.

Warm or cool: Choose the temperature that feels most comfortable and soothing on your stomach.

Stay hydrated: Aim for eight-10 glasses of water every day alongside your puréed meals.

Embrace the manual tool: Reach out to your scientific group and cherished ones for encouragement and steering.

Remember, the puréed food regimen is a temporary stepping stone in your journey. Celebrate the pass lower returned of texture, check with new flavor combinations, and accept as true with the technique as your digestive gadget prepares for the grand finale – the sector of regular food awaits!

Tropical Protein Bowl with Mashed Banana, Mango, Spinach, and Tofu Crumbles

Ingredients:

half of ripe banana, mashed

half of of cup chopped mango

1/4 cup packed sparkling spinach

1/4 cup crumbled employer tofu

1/four cup unsweetened almond milk

1 scoop vanilla protein powder

1/4 teaspoon ground cinnamon

Optional: Coconut flakes, chopped nuts

Instructions:

1.   Mash banana in a bowl.

2.   Add chopped mango, spinach, crumbled tofu, almond milk, protein powder, and cinnamon. Stir properly.

3.   Top with extra mango quantities, coconut flakes, or chopped nuts if desired.

Nutritional Information (regular with serving):

Calories: 350

Fat: 14g

Carbohydrates: 45g

Protein: 22g

Fiber: 7g

Lentil and Vegetable Soup with Coconut Milk and Turmeric

Ingredients:

1 tablespoon olive oil

1 onion, chopped

2 cloves garlic, minced

1 cup brown lentils, rinsed

four cups vegetable broth

1 cup chopped zucchini

1 cup chopped carrots

half of of of cup unsweetened coconut milk

1 teaspoon turmeric

half of teaspoon ground ginger

Salt and pepper to flavor

Instructions:

1.   Heat olive oil in a large pot over medium heat.

2.   Add onion and garlic. Cook till softened, about 5 mins.

three. Add lentils, broth, zucchini, and carrots. Bring to a boil, then reduce warmth and simmer for 20 mins, or until lentils are gentle.

four.   Stir in coconut milk, turmeric, and ginger. Simmer for a in addition 5 minutes.

five.   Season with salt and pepper to flavor.

Nutritional Information (consistent with serving):

Calories: 3 hundred, Fat: 10g, Carbohydrates: 40g, Protein: 10g, Fiber: 8g

Pumpkin Spice Chia Seed Pudding with Almond Milk

Ingredients:

1/four cup chia seeds

1 cup unsweetened almond milk

half of of of teaspoon pumpkin spice

1/4 teaspoon ground cinnamon

Pinch of nutmeg

Optional: Stevia or exceptional sweetener to taste

Instructions:

1.   Combine chia seeds, almond milk, pumpkin spice, cinnamon, and nutmeg in a jar or glass bowl. Stir properly.

2.   Cover and refrigerate in a single day.

3.   In the morning, stir yet again and alter sweetness if preferred.

four. Top with a sprinkle of pumpkin seeds or chopped nuts for brought texture and protein (non-compulsory).

Nutritional Information (in line with serving):

Calories: 250

Fat: 15g

Carbohydrates: 20g

Protein: 8g

Fiber: 8g

Berry Blast Protein Bowl with Greek Yogurt, Hemp Seeds, and Mashed Berries

Ingredients:

half of of cup simple Greek yogurt

half of of of cup mashed blended berries (which incorporates strawberries, blueberries, and raspberries)

1/4 cup hemp seeds

1 scoop vanilla protein powder

1/four teaspoon vanilla extract

Optional: Granola

Instructions:

1.   In a bowl, combine Greek yogurt, mashed berries, hemp seeds, protein powder, and vanilla extract. Stir properly.

2.   Enjoy chilled.

3.   Optional: Top with a sprinkle of granola for delivered texture and crunch.

Nutritional Information (in keeping with serving):

Calories: three hundred

Fat: 10g

Carbohydrates: 35g

Protein: 16g

Fiber: 7g

Creamy White Bean Soup with Lemon Drizzle and Fresh Herbs

Ingredients:

1 tablespoon olive oil

1 onion, chopped

2 cloves garlic, minced

1 cup cooked cannellini beans, worn-out and rinsed

4 cups vegetable broth

half of cup unsweetened coconut milk

1 lemon, juiced and zested

1/four cup sparkling parsley, chopped

Salt and pepper to taste

Instructions:

1.   Heat olive oil in a large pot over medium warmth.

2.   Add onion and garlic. Cook until softened, about 5 minutes.

3.   Add cannellini beans, broth, coconut milk, lemon juice, and zest. Bring to a boil, then reduce warmness and simmer for 15 minutes.

four. Puree soup with an immersion blender or in batches in a regular blender until clean and creamy.

five. Garnish with glowing parsley and further lemon zest if desired.

Nutritional Information (consistent with serving):

Calories: 250, Fat: 8g, Carbohydrates: 30g, Protein: 8g, Fiber: 5g

Mixed Green Protein Bowl with Avocado, Almond Milk, Protein Powder, and Spinach

Ingredients:

1 cup packed combined greens (spinach, kale, arugula)

1/2 avocado, peeled and cubed

half of cup unsweetened almond milk

1 scoop vanilla protein powder

1/four teaspoon ground cinnamon

Optional: Stevia or other sweetener to taste

Instructions:

1.   Blend all materials till easy and creamy.

2.   Adjust consistency with more almond milk if wished.

three. Enjoy chilled.

Nutritional Information (consistent with serving):

Calories: 380

Fat: 18g

Carbohydrates: 25g

Protein: 20g

Fiber: 8g

Lentil and Spinach Dal with Fresh Coriander

Ingredients:

1 tablespoon olive oil

1 onion, chopped

2 cloves garlic, minced

1 cup brown lentils, rinsed

four cups vegetable broth

1 cup chopped glowing spinach

1 (14.Five oz...) can diced tomatoes with their juices

1 teaspoon curry powder

1/2 teaspoon ground cumin

Chapter 5: Navigating the Adaptive Soft Diet Stage

You've conquered the puréed section, and now you're prepared to embody the vibrant international of easy elements!

Why the Adaptive/Soft Diet?

The adaptive/soft diet regime is a critical step to your healing approach. It introduces your digestive system to a numerous international of tender, properly-cooked, and easy-to-digest meals. This sluggish improvement guarantees cushty digestion while supplying a fulfilling and interesting dietary enjoy.

What Can You Eat?

Your menu now expands to encompass a symphony of textures and flavors:

Softly cooked greens: Steamed asparagus, roasted sweet potatoes, and gently sautéed spinach.

Well-cooked and flaked fish and hen: Baked salmon, tuna salad, or gentle-scrambled eggs for protein electricity.

Ripe culmination and greens: Sliced bananas, mashed avocado, and clean berries for an explosion of nutrients and splendor.

Whole grains and mild pastas: Cooked brown rice, quinoa porridge, or properly-cooked pasta dishes for desirable starch and fiber.

Soft cheeses and yogurt: Ricotta, mozzarella, and Greek yogurt offer protein and calcium in without issue digestible bureaucracy.

Blended smoothies and yogurt bowls: Continue playing the ones protein-packed alternatives, incorporating softer fruits and greens like bananas, mangoes, and cooked greens.

Tips for Adaptive/Soft Diet Success:

Start sluggish and concentrate for your frame: Introduce new textures often and be aware of how your stomach reacts.

Chew very well: This aids digestion and allows you revel in complete with smaller quantities.

Cook it right: Overcooked or undercooked materials may be tough to digest, so purpose for the ideal tender and succulent texture.

Portion manipulate is essential: Start with smaller food and snacks to keep away from overloading your digestive tool.

Stay hydrated: Aim for 8-10 glasses of water every day alongside your smooth food food.

Embrace the assist system: Consult your scientific institution and cherished ones for recommendation and encouragement in the route of this section.

ADAPTIVE/SOFT DIET STAGE PHASE 3

Sweet Potato and Black Bean Bisque with Cilantro Pesto

Ingredients:

1 tablespoon olive oil

1 small onion, chopped

2 cloves garlic, minced

1 huge candy potato, peeled and chopped

1 (15-ounce) can black beans, tired and rinsed

three cups vegetable broth

1/four cup chopped sparkling cilantro

1/four cup chopped walnuts

1/four cup grated Parmesan cheese

2 tablespoons olive oil

Salt and pepper to flavor

Instructions:

1.   In a big pot, warm temperature the olive oil over medium warm temperature. Add the onion and garlic and prepare dinner until the onion is softened, about five mins.

2.   Add the candy potato, black beans, and vegetable broth to the pot. Bring to a boil, then reduce the warm temperature and permit it simmer for 20 minutes or until the candy potato is easy.

3.   Use an immersion blender or transfer the soup to a blender to puree till smooth.

five.   Return the soup to the pot and keep it heat over low warmth.

6.   In a meals processor, combine the cilantro, walnuts, Parmesan cheese, and more than one tablespoons of olive oil. Pulse until a clean pesto is formed.

7.   Serve the bisque heat, garnished with the cilantro pesto.

Nutritional Information:

Calories: 220 Fat: 11g Carbohydrates: 22g Protein: 9g Fiber: 7g

Intake Recommendation: This Sweet Potato and Black Bean Bisque with Cilantro Pesto is a amazing alternative for gastric pass stage 1 patients as it is immoderate in protein and fiber, and occasional in fat. The black beans provide a fantastic supply of plant-based protein, at the equal time as the sweet potato and cilantro add flavor and crucial vitamins to the bisque.

Scrambled Tofu with Spinach and Avocado on Whole Wheat Toast

Ingredients:

1/2 block enterprise tofu, tired and crumbled

1/4 cup packed glowing spinach

1/four avocado, sliced

1 slice whole wheat toast

1 tablespoon olive oil

Salt and pepper to taste

Optional: Herbs like chives or dill

Instructions:

1.   Heat olive oil in a pan over medium warmth.

2.   Add crumbled tofu and prepare dinner till lightly browned, about 5 mins.

three. Stir in spinach and prepare dinner till wilted, about 1 minute.

4.   Season with salt and pepper to flavor.

5.   Toast the entire wheat bread.

6.   Top toast with scrambled tofu, avocado slices, and non-compulsory herbs.

Nutritional Information (consistent with serving):

Calories: three hundred, Fat: 14g, Carbohydrates: 30g. Protein: 18g, Fiber: 5g

Greek Yogurt Parfait with Mixed Berries and Granola

 Ingredients:

1 cup smooth Greek yogurt

half cup mixed berries

1/four cup granola

1 tablespoon honey (optionally available)

Instructions:

1. Layer Greek yogurt, berries, and granola in a parfait glass.

2. Drizzle with honey if favored.

3. Chill for 15 minutes earlier than gambling.

Nutritional Information (in step with serving):

Calories: 3 hundred

Fat: 10g

Carbohydrates: 40g

Protein: 15g

Fiber: 5g

Oatmeal with Chia Seeds, Berries, and Pumpkin Seeds

Chapter 6: Culinary Freedom Found

(Phase four - Month 4 and Lifelong)

You've conquered the liquid, puréed, and moderate meals ranges, and now you're prepared to embody the boundless international of ordinary components!

Why the Stabilization Diet?

The stabilization weight loss plan is a crucial step to your prolonged-time period fulfillment. It promotes aware ingesting practices, assisting you preserve a wholesome weight, optimize your dietary consumption, and revel in food with freedom and responsibility.

What Can You Eat?

The global is your oyster! You can now enjoy nearly any food, with some vital problems:

Focus on balanced nutrients: Incorporate plenty of cease result, vegetables, complete grains, lean protein, and healthful fat into your diet regime.

Portion manage is prime: Be aware about serving sizes and listen in your frame's hunger cues.

Limit horrific fats and sugars: Avoid processed components, sugary beverages, and immoderate saturated and trans fats.

Stay hydrated: Water is your excellent pal! Aim for 8-10 glasses daily.

Tips for Stabilization Diet Success:

Plan your meals and snacks: This promotes conscious ingesting and allows you keep away from awful picks.

Cook at home on every occasion viable: This offers you control over factors and element sizes.

Read meals labels: Be aware about calorie and nutrient content material cloth, specially hidden sugars and awful fats.

Move your frame: Regular bodily interest is crucial for lengthy-term weight manage and average health.

Seek help: Connect together along with your clinical physician, nutritionist, or resource business enterprise for guidance and encouragement.

Remember, the stabilization food plan is a lifelong journey. Embrace the liberty to find out new flavors and textures, and believe the method as you still nourish your body and mind.

Stabilization Diet Stage (Phase 4 - Month four and Lifelong)

High-Protein Vegetarian Entrées

Lentil Shepherd's Pie with Quinoa and Roasted Vegetables

Ingredients:

Mashed Potato Topping:

2 huge potatoes, peeled and chopped

1/2 of cup unsweetened almond milk

1 tablespoon olive oil

Salt and pepper to flavor

Lentil Stew:

1 tablespoon olive oil

1 onion, chopped

2 carrots, chopped

2 celery stalks, chopped

2 cloves garlic, minced

1 cup inexperienced lentils, rinsed

4 cups vegetable broth

1 tablespoon tomato paste

1 teaspoon dried thyme

half of of teaspoon dried rosemary

Salt and pepper to taste

Roasted Vegetables (elective):

Brussels sprouts, broccoli florets, candy potatoes, and so forth. (select out your favorites)

Instructions:

1.   Preheat oven to four hundred°F (two hundred°C).

2.   Prepare mashed potatoes: Boil potatoes till smooth, then mash with almond milk, olive oil, salt, and pepper. Set apart.

3.   Roast greens (non-obligatory): Toss determined on veggies with olive oil, salt, and pepper. Spread on a baking sheet and roast for 20-25 mins, until slight and barely browned.

4.   Make lentil stew: Heat olive oil in a huge pot or Dutch oven over medium warm temperature. Add onion, carrots, and celery. Cook till softened, approximately 5 minutes.

five.   Add garlic, lentils, broth, tomato paste, thyme, and rosemary. Bring to a boil, then reduce warmth and simmer for 20-25 minutes, or till lentils are clean. Season with salt and pepper.

6.   Assemble the shepherd's pie: Spread the lentil stew in a baking dish. Top with mashed potatoes, making peaks with a fork.

7.   Optional: Sprinkle with breadcrumbs and a drizzle of olive oil in advance than baking.

8.   Bake for 15-20 minutes, till golden brown and heated through.

Nutritional Information (in line with serving):

Calories: four   hundred,   Fat: 10g, Carbohydrates: 50g, Protein: 18g, Fiber: 10g

Tofu Stir-Fry with Brown Rice and Edamame

Ingredients:

1 tablespoon sesame oil

1 block commercial enterprise organization tofu, tired and cubed

1 bell pepper, sliced

1 broccoli floret, reduce into chew-sized portions

half of of cup sliced mushrooms

1 clove garlic, minced

1 tablespoon soy sauce

1 teaspoon rice vinegar

half of teaspoon honey

1/4 teaspoon ginger powder

1 cup cooked brown rice

half of cup frozen edamame, thawed

Instructions:

1.   Heat sesame oil in a wok or big skillet over medium-excessive heat. Add tofu and prepare dinner till golden brown on all components.

2.   Add bell pepper, broccoli, and mushrooms. Stir-fry for three-four mins, till greens are crisp-gentle.

3.   Stir in garlic, soy sauce, rice vinegar, honey, and ginger powder. Cook for 1 minute, till sauce thickens barely.

four. Serve stir-fry over brown rice and top with edamame.

Nutritional Information (in line with serving):

Calories: 350, Fat: 12g, Carbohydrates: 40g, Protein: 15g, Fiber: 5g

Black Bean Burgers on Whole Wheat Buns with Avocado and Sweet Potato Fries

Ingredients:

Black Bean Burgers:

1 (15 ounces.) can black beans, worn-out and rinsed

half of of cup rolled oats

1/4 cup chopped red onion

1/four cup chopped bell pepper

1/4 cup chopped zucchini

1 tablespoon olive oil

1 tablespoon breadcrumbs

1 teaspoon chili powder

half teaspoon cumin

Salt and pepper to taste

Hamburger Fixings:

Whole wheat buns

Avocado slices

Sliced tomato

Lettuce leaves

Optional: Onion earrings, ketchup, mustard

Sweet Potato Fries:

1 sweet potato, peeled and decrease into fries

1 tablespoon olive oil

Salt and pepper to taste

Instructions:

1.   Preheat oven to 4 hundred°F (hundred°C).

2.   Make black bean burgers: Mash black beans in a bowl. Add oats, crimson onion, bell pepper, zucchini, olive oil, breadcrumbs, chili powder, cumin, salt, and pepper. Mix well to shape patties.

3.   Place burger patties on a baking sheet and bake for 20-25 minutes, flipping halfway via cooking.

4.   Make sweet potato fries: Toss candy potato fries with olive oil, salt, and pepper. Spread on a baking sheet and bake along burgers for the final 15 mins, or till golden brown and clean.

5.   Assemble burgers on complete wheat buns collectively together with your preferred toppings. Enjoy with sweet potato fries!

Nutritional Information (steady with serving):

Calories: 500

Fat: 15g

Carbohydrates: 60g

Protein: 16g

Fiber: 10g

Vegetable Curry with Butternut Squash and Chickpeas

Ingredients:

1 tablespoon olive oil

1 onion, chopped

2 cloves garlic, minced

1 teaspoon curry powder

1/2 teaspoon ground turmeric

1/four teaspoon chili powder (optionally available)

1 (14.Five oz..) can diced tomatoes with their juices

1 cup vegetable broth

1 can (15 oz..) chickpeas, worn-out and rinsed

1 cup cubed butternut squash

1 cup chopped cauliflower, 1 bell pepper, sliced

1 cup unsweetened coconut milk

Salt and pepper to taste

Cooked brown rice or quinoa (for serving)

Instructions:

1.   Heat olive oil in a big pot or Dutch oven over medium heat. Add onion and cook dinner till softened, about five mins.

2.   Add garlic, curry powder, turmeric, and chili powder (if using). Cook for 1 minute, till aromatic.

three. Stir in tomatoes, broth, chickpeas, butternut squash, cauliflower, and bell pepper. Bring to a boil, then lessen warmness and simmer for 20-25 minutes, or till veggies are tender.

four. Stir in coconut milk and season with salt and pepper to taste. Simmer for a further 5 minutes.

5.   Serve vegetable curry over cooked brown rice or quinoa.

Stuffed Eggplant with Quinoa, Lentils, and Herbs

Ingredients:

2 eggplants, halved and seeds eliminated

1 tablespoon olive oil

1 onion, chopped

2 cloves garlic, minced

1/2 cup cooked quinoa

half of of cup cooked brown lentils

half of cup chopped tomatoes

1/4 cup chopped sparkling parsley

1/4 cup chopped sparkling mint

1 teaspoon lemon juice

Salt and pepper to taste

Instructions:

1.   Preheat oven to four hundred°F (hundred°C).

2.   Brush the inner of the eggplants with olive oil and sprinkle with salt and pepper. Place them on a baking sheet, reduce-thing down, and roast for 15 minutes.

three. While the eggplants roast, warmth olive oil in a skillet over medium warmth. Add onion and cook dinner dinner till softened, approximately five minutes.

four. Add garlic and cook dinner dinner dinner for a in addition minute.

five. Stir in cooked quinoa, lentils, tomatoes, parsley, mint, and lemon juice. Season with salt and pepper to flavor.

6.   Once the eggplants are roasted, fill them with the quinoa combination.

7.   Bake for a in addition 10-15 mins, until heated via.

Tofu Scramble with Spinach and Mushrooms on Whole Wheat Toast

Ingredients:

1 block corporation tofu, worn-out and crumbled

1 tablespoon olive oil

1/2 of onion, chopped

2 cloves garlic, minced

1 cup chopped spinach

1/2 of cup sliced mushrooms

1/4 teaspoon turmeric

Salt and pepper to taste

2 slices entire wheat toast

Instructions:

1.   Heat olive oil in a skillet over medium heat. Add onion and cook dinner until softened, approximately five minutes.

2.   Add garlic and put together dinner for a similarly minute.

3.   Stir in crumbled tofu and cook dinner dinner for five-7 mins, breaking it up with a spatula.

4.   Add spinach and mushrooms and prepare dinner dinner until wilted and mild.

5.   Stir in turmeric and season with salt and pepper to flavor.

6.   Toast the entire wheat bread.

7.   Serve the tofu scramble on pinnacle of the toast.

Chapter 7: Roasted Tomatoes and Avocado

Ingredients:

1/4 cup chickpea flour

1/4 cup water

1/4 teaspoon turmeric

Salt and pepper to flavor

1 tablespoon olive oil

1/2 of cup chopped spinach

1/four cup crumbled goat cheese (optionally available)

1 sliced tomato, roasted within the oven (optionally available)

1/four sliced avocado

Instructions:

1.   Preheat oven to four hundred°F (2 hundred°C) if the usage of roasted tomatoes. Place sliced tomato on a baking sheet, drizzle

with olive oil, and roast for 15-20 mins until barely softened.

2.   In a bowl, whisk collectively chickpea flour, water, turmeric, salt, and pepper. Let the batter sit down down down for 5 mins to thicken.

3.   Heat olive oil in a non-stick pan over medium warm temperature. Pour within the chickpea batter and swirl to coat the lowest of the pan.

4.   Cook for 2-three mins, or till the edges start to set.

five.   Add spinach and put together dinner dinner for any other minute, until wilted.

6.   Sprinkle with goat cheese (if using) and fold the omelette in half.

7.   Slide the omelette onto a plate and top with roasted tomato slices and avocado. Enjoy!

Roasted Broccoli with Garlic and Lemon Zest

Ingredients:

1 head of broccoli, reduce into florets

1 tablespoon olive oil

1 clove garlic, minced

half of of teaspoon dried oregano

Salt and pepper to taste

Zest of 1/2 lemon

Instructions:

1.	Preheat oven to 4 hundred°F (hundred°C).

2.	Toss broccoli florets with olive oil, garlic, oregano, salt, and pepper.

3.	Spread broccoli on a baking sheet in a unmarried layer.

four.	Roast for 15-20 minutes, or until mild and slightly browned.

five.	Sprinkle with lemon zest in advance than serving.

Nutritional Information (in step with serving):

Calories: 70

Fat: 4g

Carbohydrates: 7g

Protein: 3g

Fiber: 3g

Quinoa Salad with Chopped Vegetables and Tahini Dressing

Ingredients:

1 cup cooked quinoa

half of cup chopped cucumber

1/2 of cup chopped tomatoes

1/4 cup chopped purple onion

1/four cup chopped clean parsley

2 tablespoons tahini

1 tablespoon lemon juice

1 teaspoon water

1/4 teaspoon ground cumin

Salt and pepper to flavor

Instructions:

1. Cook quinoa steady with bundle instructions. Let cool.

2. In a big bowl, integrate cooked quinoa, cucumber, tomatoes, purple onion, and parsley.

3. Whisk together tahini, lemon juice, water, cumin, salt, and pepper to make the dressing.

four. Pour the dressing over the quinoa aggregate and toss to coat.

5. Chill for at the least half-hour earlier than serving.

Nutritional Information (regular with serving): Calories: 250

Fat: 8g

Carbohydrates: 35g

Protein: 8g, Fiber: 5g

Steamed Green Beans with Almonds and Sesame Seeds

Ingredients:

1 cup inexperienced beans, trimmed

1/four cup sliced almonds

1 tablespoon sesame seeds

1 tablespoon low-sodium soy sauce

1 teaspoon rice vinegar

half of teaspoon honey

Instructions:

1.   Bring a pot of water to a boil.

2.   Add inexperienced beans and steam for three-4 minutes, or till moderate-crisp.

three. While the beans are steaming, warm temperature a small skillet over medium warmness.

four. Add almonds and toast till golden brown, approximately three minutes.

five. In a bowl, whisk collectively soy sauce, rice vinegar, and honey.

6. Toss steamed inexperienced beans with the sauce, toasted almonds, and sesame seeds.

7. Serve at once.

Nutritional Information (regular with serving):

Calories: one hundred fifty, Fat: 8g, Carbohydrates: 15g, Protein: 4g, Fiber: 3g

Mashed Sweet Potato with Cinnamon and Maple Syrup

Ingredients:

1 large sweet potato, peeled and chopped

1/four cup water

1/four teaspoon floor cinnamon

1 tablespoon maple syrup (non-compulsory)

Instructions:

1.   Place sweet potato and water in a saucepan and produce to a boil.

2.   Reduce warmness and simmer for 15-20 minutes, or till moderate.

three. Drain any greater water.

4.   Mash sweet potato with cinnamon and maple syrup (if the use of).

five.   Serve warmth.

Nutritional Information (steady with serving):

Chapter 8: Hummus and Vegetable Crudités

Ingredients:

1/4 cup hummus

Assorted uncooked vegetables like carrots, cucumber, bell pepper, celery, broccoli florets

Instructions:

1.   Scoop hummus right right right into a small bowl.

2.   Arrange your chosen uncooked vegetables across the hummus dip.

three. Enjoy the crunchy goodness!

Nutritional Information (constant with serving):

Calories: one hundred and 80

Fat: 5g

Carbohydrates: 20g

Protein: 7g

Fiber: 5g

Greek Yogurt with Granola and Berries

Ingredients:

1/2 of of cup undeniable Greek yogurt

1/four cup unsweetened granola

1/four cup blended berries (blackberries, blueberries, raspberries)

Instructions:

1.   Spoon Greek yogurt proper right into a small bowl.

2.   Sprinkle with granola and berries.

three. Mix and get pride from the creamy sweetness!

Nutritional Information (in line with serving):

Calories: two hundred

Fat: 5g

Carbohydrates: 25g

Protein: 12g

Fiber: 3g

Edamame pods with sea salt

Ingredients:

1 cup frozen edamame pods, thawed

Instructions:

1.   Thaw frozen edamame pods under bloodless on foot water or inside the microwave.

2.   Sprinkle with sea salt (non-compulsory) and experience the protein-packed pop!

Nutritional Information (in keeping with serving):

Calories: a hundred and eighty

Fat: 5g

Carbohydrates: 15g

Protein: 8g

Fiber: 4g

Apple slices with almond butter

Ingredients:

1 apple, sliced

1 tablespoon almond butter

Instructions:

1.   Slice your apple into chew-sized portions.

2.   Spread almond butter on each slice.

3.   Savor the candy and nutty aggregate!

Nutritional Information (consistent with serving):

Calories: 100 fifty

Fat: 5g

Carbohydrates: 20g

Protein: 5g

Fiber: 4g

Roasted chickpeas with spices

Ingredients:

1 cup dried chickpeas, rinsed and drained

1 tablespoon olive oil

half of of teaspoon paprika

1/four teaspoon cumin

Salt and pepper to taste

Instructions:

1.   Preheat oven to 4 hundred°F (hundred°C).

2.   Toss chickpeas with olive oil, spices, and salt and pepper.

three. Spread on a baking sheet and roast for 20-25 minutes, or until golden brown and crispy.

four.   Enjoy the spiced, crunchy snack!

Nutritional Information (in step with serving):

Calories: two hundred

Fat: 5g

Carbohydrates: 20g

Protein: 6g

Fiber: 5g

Chapter 9: Breakfast Recipes

1. Carrot, Apple and Ginger Juice

Preparation Time: 10 minutes

Cooking Time: zero mins

Servings: 2

Ingredients:

4 carrots peeled and shape of chopped

1 apple cored and sort of chopped

1 tablespoon grated ginger

½ lemon, juiced

1 cup water

6 mint leaves, more or a lot much less chopped

Directions:

Place all substances, except lemon juice, in a blender and puree.

Strain the puree through a first rate sieve to make the juice and discard the pulp.

Add the lemon juice and stir. If you need a terrific thinner juice, you can dilute it with clean water. Serve and enjoy.

Nutrition: Calories: 78 - Fat: 0 g - Protein: 1 g - Carbs: 16 g - Sugar: 12 g - Fiber: 2 g

2. Berries Parfait and Greek Yogurt

Preparation Time: 5 minutes

Cooking Time: zero mins

Servings: 2

Ingredients:

1 cup non-fat clean Greek yogurt

¼ cup sparkling strawberries

¼ cup easy raspberries

¼ cup glowing cranberries

1 tablespoon walnuts, chopped

1 teaspoon agave nectar

Directions:

Chop the strawberries.

In two glasses layer yogurt, strawberries, cranberries and raspberries.

Top with walnuts and agave nectar

SUGGESTION: walnuts can be too difficult for the early levels of restoration. If you do not tolerate walnuts, or the extent of your diet plan ought to now not call for them, without a doubt dispose of them from the recipe.

Nutrition: Calories: 245 - Fat: 11 g - Protein: 16 g - Carbs: 25 g - Fiber: five g - Sugar: 21 g - Sodium: 46 g

3. Italian Style Tomatoes and Scrambled Eggs

Preparation Time: 5 mins

Cooking Time: forty five minutes

Servings: 2

Ingredients:

3 eggs

eight oz... No-salt delivered canned tomatoes, diced

½ white onion, diced

1 tablespoon sparkling basil, chopped

1 teaspoon dried thyme

Sea salt and pepper

Cooking spray

Directions:

In a skillet, warm temperature spayed olive oil on medium.

When oil is warm, stir inside the onion and sauté for approximately 5 mins, or until it's golden.

Low the warmth and upload tomatoes and thyme, simmering for 30-35 mins, until tomatoes begin to form a thickened sauce.

In a bowl, whisk the eggs with salt and pepper; then, upload to the tomato and cook dinner over medium warmness, stirring to combine.

When the eggs are set and soft, dispose of from heat, sprinkle with basil, and serve.

Nutrition: Calories: 241 - Fat: 14 g - Protein: 13 g - Carbs: 12 g - Sodium: 148 mg

four. Mexican Scrambled Eggs

Preparation Time: 10 mins

Cooking Time: 15 minutes

Servings: 2

Ingredients:

2 eggs, lightly overwhelmed

1 tomato, diced

½ small purple bell pepper, diced

2 tablespoons onion, finely chopped

1 cup no-salt introduced black beans, tired and rinsed

2 tablespoons low-fats Mexican cheese, shredded

1 tablespoon olive oil

½ teaspoon cumin

½ teaspoon paprika

1 tablespoon glowing parsley, chopped

A pinch sea salt

A pinch black pepper

Directions:

In a big skillet, warm temperature oil over medium warmth.

Add onion and put together dinner until aromatic for about 2-3 mins. Then, stir in pink bell pepper and put together dinner for 3 mins earlier than such as the tomato and black beans, cumin and paprika. Continue stirring and cook dinner for two-three mins greater.

While veggies are cooking, whisk the eggs and season with salt and pepper.

Add eggs to the skillet, and keep to prepare dinner dinner, at the same time as stirring, until nearly set and clean for about 2 minutes.

When eggs are nearly completed, upload cheese and keep cooking for approximately 1 minute till the cheese melts. Sprinkle with parsley, serve and experience.

Nutrition: Calories: 229 - Total fat: 15 g - Protein: 14 g - Carbs: 12 g - Sodium: 149 mg

5. Spinach and Mushrooms Omelet

Preparation Time: 10 mins

Cooking Time: 10 mins

Servings: 2

Ingredients:

½ cup spinach, chopped

½ cup mushrooms, sliced

2 tablespoons white onion, diced

2 eggs

1 teaspoon garlic powder

½ teaspoon sea salt

¼ teaspoon ground black pepper

Cooking spray

Directions:

Lightly grease a skillet with cooking spray over medium warmth.

Cook onion for about 2-three minutes; then add garlic powder and mushrooms, stirring continuously.

Cook for 3 minutes and stir inside the spinach until wilts. Meanwhile, whisk the eggs, seasoning with salt and pepper.

When the mushrooms and vegetables combination is ready, pour eggs inside the skillet and coat flippantly the combination.

Cook till the eggs are set, and fold the omelet in half of.

Remove from warmth, reduce in 1/2 and serve.

Nutrition: Calories: 232 - Fat: thirteen g - Protein: 21 g - Carbs: 3 g - Sodium: 336 mg

6. Almond Protein Porridge

Preparation Time: 5 minutes

Cooking Time: 25 mins

Servings: 1

Ingredients:

¼ cup uncooked steel lessen oats

¾ cup low-fat milk

1 tablespoon all-natural creamy almond butter

1 tablespoon no-sugar introduced raisins

1 tablespoon chia seeds

½ banana, sliced

1 scoop protein powder (optionally to be had)

Directions:

In a saucepan over immoderate heat, deliver the milk to a boil.

Add the oats and raisins. Low the heat and simmer for 20 mins, stirring frequently.

When the oats have thickened, do away with from the warm temperature.

Let the aggregate rest for 1 minute. Stir in protein powder (if using).

Top with the banana slices, almond butter and chia seeds. Enjoy warm temperature.

Nutrition: Calories: 295 - Fat: 14 g - Protein: 10 g - Carbs: 28 g - Fiber: 7 g - Sugar: 10 g

7. Summer Breakfast Quinoa Bowls

Preparation Time: five minutes

Cooking Time: 20 minutes

Servings: 2

Ingredients:

1 sliced peach

1/three c. Quinoa

1 c. Low-fat milk

½ tsp. Vanilla extract

2 tsps. Natural stevia

12 raspberries

14 blueberries

2 tsps. Honey

Directions:

Add natural stevia, 2/three c. Milk, and quinoa to a saucepan, and stir to combine.

Over medium-immoderate warmness, carry to a boil, then cowl and reduce heat to a low simmer for a similarly 20 minutes (you have to be capable of fluff quinoa with a fork).

Grease and preheat grill to medium. Grill peach slices for approximately a minute steady with aspect. Set apart.

Heat ultimate milk in the microwave and set apart.

Split cooked quinoa flippantly among 2 serving bowls and pinnacle gently with final elements. Enjoy!

Nutrition: Carbs 36 g Fats four g Sugar 3 g Calories one hundred and 80

eight. Very Berry Muesli

Preparation Time: 6 hours

Cooking Time: zero mins

Servings: 2

Ingredients:

1 c. Oats

1 c. Fruit-flavored yogurt

½ c. Milk

1/eight tsp. Salt

½ c. Dried raisins

½ c. Chopped apple

½ c. Frozen blueberries

¼ c. Chopped walnuts

Directions:

Combine yogurt, salt and oats in a medium bowl, combo properly and then cover the aggregate tightly.

Place in the refrigerator to cool for six hours.

Add raisins and apples the gently fold.

Top with walnuts and serve. Enjoy!

Nutrition: Carbs 31.2 g Fats four.Three g Sugar 3 g Calories 198

nine. Watermelon Mint Infused Water

Preparation Time: 10 minutes

Cooking Time: zero mins

Servings: 4

Ingredients:

Mint leaves (8)

Water (4 c.)

Sliced watermelon (1.Five c)

Directions:

Add all of the elements into a pitcher jar and stir round.

Place into the fridge to set for about an hour in advance than serving.

Nutrition: Calories 25 Carbs 6g Fat zero.3g Protein 1.2g

10. Strawberry & Mushroom Breakfast Sandwich

Preparation Time: 10 mins

Cooking Time: 0 mins

Servings: 1

Ingredients:

three ounces.. Cream cheese

1 tbsp. Honey

1 tbsp. Grated Lemon zest

four sliced Portobello Mushrooms

2 c. Sliced Strawberries

Directions:

Add honey, lemon zest, and cheese to a meals processor and way till truly blanketed.

Use cheese combination to unfold on mushrooms as you will butter.

Top with strawberries. Enjoy!

Nutrition: Carbs 6 g Fats 6 g Sugar 2 g Calories 100 80

11. Summer Breakfast Quinoa Bowls

Preparation Time: five mins

Cooking Time: 20 minutes

Servings: 2

Ingredients:

1 sliced peach

1/three c. Quinoa

1 c. Low-fats milk

½ tsp. Vanilla extract

2 tsps. Natural stevia

12 raspberries

14 blueberries

2 tsps. Honey

Directions:

Add herbal stevia, 2/three c. Milk and quinoa to a saucepan, and stir to mix.

Over medium-immoderate warmth, supply to a boil then cover and decrease warmth to a low simmer for a in addition 20 minutes (you ought so you can fluff quinoa with a fork).

Grease and preheat grill to medium. Grill peach slices for approximately a minute constant with thing. Set aside.

Heat very last milk within the microwave and set apart.

Split cooked quinoa evenly among 2 serving bowls and top evenly with very last elements. Enjoy!

Nutrition: Carbs 36 g Fats 4 g Sugar 3 g Calories a hundred eighty

12. Beef Purée

Preparation time: half of of-hour

Cooking time: four to 10 hours

Servings: four

Ingredients:

1 pound (454 g) pork tenderloin steak

1 teaspoon olive oil

1 teaspoon soy sauce

½ teaspoon salt, plus greater to flavor

½ teaspoon garlic powder

½ teaspoon onion powder

½ teaspoon dried rosemary, crushed

½ teaspoon dried parsley

¼ teaspoon freshly ground black pepper, plus greater to taste

Beef inventory, as wanted

Directions:

Pat the steak dry with paper towels and brush with olive oil and soy sauce. Mix salt, garlic powder, onion powder, rosemary, parsley and pepper and rub over steak. Cook the steak in a gradual cooker until cooked through and the internal temperature reaches 145ºF (63ºC), 8 to ten hours on the low putting or four to 5 hours at the excessive setting.

Remove the steak from sluggish cooker, reserving the cooking juices. Put the steak in a included subject and refrigerate until chilled through, approximately 2 hours.

Cut the chilled steak into 1-inch cubes. Put approximately 1 cup steak cubes in a food processor and pulse until great and powdery. Add approximately ¼ cup reserved cooking juices plus stock as needed and device until clean. Repeat with very last steak cubes.

Season the puréed steak with salt and pepper and stir till very well mixed.

Serve right away.

Nutrition: electricity normal carbs: 1g universal fats: 7.9g zero fiber: zero sodium: 410mg

13. Blueberry and Spinach Smoothie

Preparation time: 5 mins

Cooking time: 2 mins

Servings: 4

Ingredients:

2 cups blueberries

three cups chopped clean spinach

½ cup chopped smooth coriander

Juice of one lemon

1-inch smooth ginger, grated

2 cups water

Directions:

Put all the materials within the blender, pulse for two minutes or till easy.

Serve immediately.

Nutrition: strength: 121 preferred carbs: 30.0g good sized fats: zero.6g half of-hour

Cooking time: 10 minutes

Servings: 6

Ingredients:

1 pound(454 g) sparkling broccoli, reduce into florets

½ cup water

½ teaspoon salt, plus extra to taste

1 teaspoon butter

1 teaspoon lemon juice

½ teaspoon onion powder

Freshly floor black pepper, to taste

Directions:

Mix the broccoli florets, water and ½ teaspoon salt in a medium saucepan and bring to a simmer. Reduce warm temperature, cover the pan and simmer until the broccoli is smooth, 5 to 10 mins.

Drain the broccoli, booking the cooking water. Add the butter, lemon juice and onion powder, season with salt and pepper and permit cool.

Put about 1 cup broccoli florets and ¼ cup cooking water in a food processor and pulse until easy. Repeal with last broccoli.

Serve immediately.

Nutrition: power overall carbs: four.3g simple fats: 0.9g minutes

Cooking Time: half-hour

Servings: 1

Ingredients:

¼ c. Canola oil

4 tbsps. Honey

1½ tsp. Vanilla

6 c. Old college rolled oats

1 c. Almond

½ c. Shredded unsweetened coconut

2 c. Bran flakes

three/four c. Chopped walnuts

1 c. Raisins

Cooking spray

Directions:

Prepare oven to preheat at 325 degrees F.

In a saucepan, put together dinner oil and vanilla gently over low flame, on occasion stirring for form of 5 minutes.

Place all elements except raisins right right into a massive bowl and combine.

Stir in honey and oil mixture slowly, ensuring all grains are properly blanketed.

Set a parchment paper on the baking tray or use cooking spray to oil lightly. Spread cereal evenly inside the tray and bake for 25 minutes, occasionally stirring to hold the mixture from burning, or till very lightly browned.

When prepared, get rid of cereal and positioned it apart to loosen up.

Add raisins and blend well.

Nutrition: Carbs sixty two g Fats 7 g Sugar 3 g Calories 458

16. Pumpkin Smoothie

Preparation time: 5 mins.

Cooking time: zero mins.

Servings: 2

Ingredients:

½ cup pumpkin purée

4 Medjool dates, pitted and chopped

1 cup unsweetened almond milk

¼ teaspoon vanilla extract

¼ teaspoon ground cinnamon

½ cup ice

A pinch of ground nutmeg

Directions:

Add all of the additives to a blender, then method till the mixture is glossy and nicely combined.

Serve without delay.

Nutrition: Calories: 417 Fat: 3g Carbs: ninety 4.9g Fiber: 10.4g Protein: eleven.4g

17. Super Smoothie

Preparation time: five minutes.

Cooking time: 0 mins.

Servings: 2

Ingredients:

1 Avocado, peeled

1 cup chopped mango

1 cup raspberries

¼ cup rolled oats

1 carrot, peeled

1 cup chopped smooth kale

2 tablespoons chopped clean parsley

1 tablespoon flaxseeds

1 tablespoon grated clean ginger

½ cup unsweetened soy milk

1 cup water

Directions:

Put all of the materials in a food processor, then blitz until sleek and clean.

Serve right now or relax inside the fridge for 1 hour in advance than serving.

Nutrition: Calories: 550 Fat: 39g Carbs: 31g Fiber: 15g Protein: 13g

Chapter 10: Lunch Recipes

21. Potato and Broccoli Soup

Preparation Time: 10 mins

Cooking Time: 20 mins

Servings: 2

Ingredients:

1 cup broccoli, chopped

1 small potato, cooked and chopped

½ onion, diced

1 garlic clove, minced

1 cup low-sodium vegetable broth

2 tablespoons Parmesan cheese, grated

1 tablespoon extra-virgin olive oil

1 teaspoon red pepper flakes

1 teaspoon turmeric

1 teaspoon sea salt

Directions:

In a small pot over medium-excessive heat, supply water to a boil.

Add in the broccoli and salt and prepare dinner for three-four minutes. Drain and set apart.

Heat the oil in a saucepan over medium warmth.

Stir inside the onion and garlic and cook dinner dinner until golden.

Add the broccoli, pink pepper flakes and potato, and put together dinner for 3 minutes.

Pour inside the broth and convey to a boil.

Remove from warmth, switch the potato and broccoli to a mixer, upload the turmeric, and pulse till puréed.

Divide into soup plates, pinnacle with Parmesan cheese and serve.

Nutrition: Calories: 271 - Fat: 7 g - Protein: 11 g - Carbs: 32 g - Sugar: 4 g - Fiber: 5 g - Sodium: 421 mg

22. Mint and Yogurt Creamy Zucchini Soup

Preparation Time: 10 mins

Cooking Time: 25 minutes

Servings: 2

Ingredients:

2 zucchinis, chopped

½ celery stalk, chopped

1 shallot, sliced

1 carrot, diced

1 tablespoon more-virgin olive oil

2 cups low-sodium vegetable broth

½ cup no-sugar added soy milk

2 tablespoons low-fats simple Greek yogurt

2 teaspoons smooth mint, minced

1 teaspoon chili powder

A pinch sea salt

A pinch black pepper

Directions:

Heat the oil in a soup pot over medium warm temperature.

Add the shallot, and put together dinner till aromatic for about 2 minutes.

Stir inside the carrot and celery, and preserve cooking for each other 2-3 minutes.

Add the zucchinis, chili powder and salt, and prepare dinner for approximately three mins, stirring continuously.

Pour in the broth, decrease the warm temperature and simmer for 15 mins, or till the zucchinis are smooth.

Add pepper, stir well, and, the use of an immersion blender, mixture until smooth.

Stir within the soy milk, and put together dinner for 1 minute extra.

Divide into soup plates, pinnacle with Greek yogurt and scatter with mint.

Nutrition: Calories: 244 - Fat: 13 g - Protein: 4 g - Carbs: 14 g - Sugar: 10 g - Fiber: 2 g - Sodium: 491 mg

23. Carrot, Zucchini and Leeks Purée

Preparation Time: 10 minute

Cooking Time: 25 minutes

Servings: four-6

Ingredients:

1 leek, stems removed and form of chopped

3. Carrots, chopped

1 zucchini, chopped

1 cup low-sodium vegetable broth, warmed

1 tablespoon Parmesan cheese, grated

1 tablespoon more-virgin olive oil

A pinch black pepper

A pinch sea salt

Water

Directions:

Over medium heat, deliver a pot of salted water to a boil.

Add the leeks and the carrots and prepare dinner for about 10 mins. Then, add the zucchini and put together dinner for 5 mins more. Drain and set aside.

In a saucepan over medium warmth, add the oil and stir within the vegetables, cooking for 1-2 minutes.

Pour in the broth and cook dinner dinner for four-5 mins, or until maximum of the broth has been absorbed. Transfer to a mixer and pulse until clean.

Return the aggregate inside the saucepan over low warmth, add Parmesan and black pepper, stir well, and serve warm.

Nutrition: Calories: 162 - Fat: 4 g - Protein: four g - Carbs: 20 g - Sodium: 376 mg

24. Cauliflower Purée

Preparation Time: five mins

Cooking Time: 15-20 minutes

Servings: 1

Ingredients:

four oz... Frozen cauliflower or glowing cauliflower, coarsely chopped

¼ cup low-sodium vegetable broth

A pinch sea salt

A pinch black pepper

A pinch nutmeg

6 cups water

Directions:

In a small saucepan pour water, upload cauliflower, black pepper and salt, and prepare dinner dinner for approximately 15 mins. Cauliflower ought to become gentle.

After cooking, drain cauliflower from extra water and pat it dry with paper towel.

Mash the cooked cauliflower. Add the broth and nutmeg into the mashed cauliflower, stir, and put together dinner dinner till broth is absorbed. Serve heat.

Nutrition: Calories: a hundred sixty 5 - Fat: 4 g - Carbs: 23 g - Protein: 6 g - Sodium: 318 mg

25. Puréed Tuna with Chives

Preparation Time: 5 minutes

Cooking Time: zero mins

Servings: 2

Ingredients:

four ounces.. Canned tuna in water, tired

2 tablespoons low-fats cream cheese

1 teaspoon lemon juice

2 teaspoons chives, chopped

A pinch white pepper

Directions:

Add all of the additives in a mixer and technique until smooth and creamy.

Nutrition: Calories: eighty - Fat: 3.Five g - Protein: 12 g - Carbs: 2 g - Cholesterol: 18 mg - Sugar: 1.Five g - Sodium: a hundred mg

26. Yogurt Salmon Paté

Preparation Time: five mins

Cooking Time: 0 minutes

Servings: 1

Ingredients:

2 ounces.. Canned salmon in water, worn-out

1 tablespoon low-fat simple Greek yogurt

1 teaspoon sparkling parsley, chopped

½ teaspoon balsamic vinegar

A pinch purple pepper

Directions:

Add all the factors in a food processor and blend until smooth and well mixed.

Nutrition: Calories: eighty two - Fat: 6 g - Protein: 11 g - Carbs: 1 g - Sugar: 2 g - Sodium: 118 mg

27. Creamy Broccoli Soup

Preparation Time: 10 mins

Cooking Time: 15 minutes

Servings: 6-eight

Ingredients:

4 cups broccoli, chopped

2 cups low-sodium vegetable inventory

1 purple bell pepper, chopped

1 avocado, more or less chopped

2 onions, chopped

2 celery stalks, sliced

Sea salt and black pepper, as needed

Ground ginger, to taste

Water

2 tablespoons smooth parsley, chopped

Directions:

Over medium heat, deliver water to a boil in a small pot.

Add broccoli and season with salt to taste. Lower the warmth and simmer for 10 mins.

Drain the broccoli and switch to a blender with bell pepper, avocado, onions, black pepper, and celery stalks.

Add broth a piece at a time to attain favored consistency, and mix until smooth.

Return the cream to the pot and cook dinner dinner over low-medium warmth for approximately 1 minute, or till heated thru.

Serve with ginger on your liking. Garnish with parsley. Enjoy.

Nutrition: Calories: 236 - Fat: eleven g - Protein: eleven g - Carbs: 17 g - Fiber: four g

28. Soft Celery Soup

Preparation Time: five minutes

Cooking Time: 10 mins

Servings: 2

Ingredients:

5 celery stalks, chopped

three cups low-sodium vegetable stock

3 tablespoons almonds, finely chopped

Sea salt and pepper, to taste

Directions:

Add stock in a saucepan and produce to boil over excessive warmness.

Add celery and cook dinner for 8 mins.

Remove from warmth and using immersion blender purée till clean.

Add almonds and stir well. Season with pepper and salt. Serve and experience.

SUGGESTION: use chopped almonds great if the level of your weight loss program and recuperation permits it; otherwise skip over them. Soup stays brilliant!

Nutrition: Calories: 104 - Fat: 6 g - Protein: four g - Carbs: 15 g - Fiber: 4 g - Sugar: 2 g

29. Cauliflower Smooth Soup

Preparation Time: 10 mins

Cooking Time: 25 mins

Servings: 2

Ingredients:

½ head cauliflower, chopped

2 garlic cloves, minced

15 ounces.. Low-sodium vegetable inventory

½ onion, diced

1 tablespoon olive oil

¼ teaspoon pepper

½ teaspoon sea salt

Directions:

Heat oil in a saucepan over medium warm temperature. Add onion and garlic and sauté for 4-five mins.

Add cauliflower and inventory, and stir well. Bring to a boil.

Reduce the warm temperature to low, cowl and simmer for 15 minutes. Season with pepper and salt.

Purée the soup the use of an immersion blender till smooth. Serve and experience.

Nutrition: Calories: 113 - Fat: eleven g - Protein: 4 g - Carbs: 14 g - Fiber: 5 g - Sugar: five g

30. Pork, White Bean, and Kale Soup

Preparation Time: 10 mins

Cooking Time: 45 mins

Servings: 6-eight

Ingredients:

2 (4 oz.) boneless beef chops, lessen into 1 inch cubes

1 (15 ounces..) can super northern beans, drained and rinsed

8 oz. Clean kale leaves

1 (14.Five oz....) can tomatoes, diced

1 teaspoon more-virgin olive oil

1 medium onion, chopped

three cups low-sodium fowl broth

½ teaspoon dried thyme

½ teaspoon dried sage

1 ½ teaspoon smoked paprika

¼ teaspoon crimson pepper flakes, overwhelmed

Directions:

Place a huge soup pot or Dutch oven over medium heat and heat the olive oil.

Add the onion and sauté for 2-3 mins, or till easy.

Add the pork and brown it for 4-5 mins on every aspect.

Mix inside the tomatoes, broth, thyme, sage, paprika, pink pepper flakes and beans, and bring to a boil.

Lower the heat and simmer, covered, for half-hour.

Add the kale and stir till wilted, approximately five mins. Serve right now.

Nutrition: Calories: 196 - Fat: five g - Protein: 18 g - Carbs: 17 g - Fiber: 6 g - Sugar: 4 g - Sodium: 581 mg

31. Apple Peanut Butter Shake

Preparation Time: 5 minutes

Cooking Time: five minutes

Servings: 1

Ingredients:

half of apple, peel and diced

2 tbsp. Peanut powder

three/four c. Ice

1 scoop chocolate protein powder

oz.. Unsweetened almond milk

Directions:

Add all components into the blender and blend until easy and creamy.

Serve and revel in.

Nutrition: Calories 203 Fat 1.Five g Carbohydrates 14 g Sugar 8 g Protein 32.Five g

32. Celery Soup

Preparation Time: 18 mins

Cooking Time: 10 mins

Servings: 2

Ingredients:

five celery stalks, chopped

three cups vegetable inventory

3 tbsp. Almonds, chopped

Pepper

Salt

Directions:

Add inventory in a saucepan and bring to boil over immoderate warmth for two

minutes.

Add celery and prepare dinner for eight mins.

Remove from warmness and using immersion blender puree until smooth.

Add almonds and stir properly.

Season with pepper and salt.

Serve and experience.

Nutrition: Calories 80 Fat 6 g Carbohydrates 5 g Sugar 2 g Protein three g

33. Vanilla Strawberry Milkshake

Preparation Time: five minutes

Cooking Time: five minutes

Servings: 1

Ingredients:

half of c. Fresh strawberries

1 c. Unsweetened almond milk

half tsp vanilla

1 tbsp. Coconut oil

1/4 c. Coconut milk

6 drops liquid stevia

Directions:

Add all factors into the blender and mix till easy and creamy.

Serve and revel in.

Nutrition: Calories 315 Fat 3 g Carbohydrates 10.6 g Sugar 5 g Protein 2.6 g

Chapter 11: Dinner Recipes

37. Two Mushrooms Soup

Preparation Time: 15 minutes

Cooking Time: 25 minutes

Servings: 2

Ingredients:

1 ¼ cup sparkling Portobello mushrooms, sliced

1 ¼ cup clean button mushrooms, sliced

½ cup white onion, chopped

2 teaspoons avocado oil

1 garlic clove, overwhelmed

½ teaspoon dried thyme

1 ¾ cup unsweetened coconut milk

1 ½ cup spring water

A pinch sea salt

A pinch cayenne powder

Directions:

In a soup pan, warmth the avocado oil over medium-excessive warmth.

Add the mushrooms, onion, garlic, thyme, salt and cayenne powder, and prepare dinner for approximately 5-6 mins. Then, take away garlic clove.

Add in the coconut milk and water and bring to a boil.

Now, modify the warm temperature to medium-low and simmer for about 10-15 mins, stirring now and again. Serve heat.

Nutrition: Calories: 177 - Fat: thirteen g - Protein: 3 g - Carbs: 6 g - Fiber: 1 g

38. Apple Cinnamon Oatmeal

Preparation Time: 10 minutes

Cooking Time: 10 minutes

Servings: 2

Ingredients:

1 cup rolled oats

2 cups water

1 cup apple, diced small

¼ teaspoon cinnamon

½ tablespoon calorie-unfastened sweetener (non-compulsory)

Directions:

In a saucepan upload oats, apple, water and cinnamon, and produce to a boil over medium warm temperature.

When it's boiling decrease warmth to low and prepare dinner dinner until oats and apple turn out to be clean.

Remove from warm temperature and flavor: if the apples did now not sweeten the oats enough, add sweetener. Otherwise, serve and enjoy.

Nutrition: Calories: a hundred thirty - Fat: 1 g - Protein: 4 g - Carbs: 23 g - Sodium: 176 mg - Fiber: 4 g - Sugar: 6 g

39. Banana Strawberries Oatmeal with Almond Butter

Preparation Time: 5 mins

Cooking Time: 10 minutes

Servings: 2

Ingredients:

1 cup rolled oats

1 cup unsweetened almond milk

10 sparkling or frozen strawberries, cored and sliced

1 banana, peeled and mashed

¼ teaspoon liquid stevia

1 teaspoon vanilla extract

⅓ teaspoon ground cinnamon

A pinch sea salt

6 massive egg whites

2 tablespoons herbal almond butter

½ cup water

Directions:

In a medium bowl, whisk egg whites and stevia, and set aside.

Over medium-immoderate warmth, in a pot, heat oats, almond milk, water, strawberries, banana, cinnamon, vanilla, and salt.

When boiling, lower the warm temperature and prepare dinner stirring on occasion for approximately 4-five mins, till the mixture is kind of set and the maximum of the beverages is absorbed.

Add the egg whites to cooked cereal and stir fast until consistency is prepared and soft.

Divide oatmeal in bowls, top with almond butter and revel in.

Nutrition: Calories: 312 - Fat: 13 g - Protein: 17 g - Carbs: 45 g - Sugar: 19 g

40. Chocolate Almond Ginger Mousse

Preparation Time: 3 hours to loosen up

Cooking Time: 0 minutes

Servings: 6

Ingredients:

1 ⅓ cup unsweetened almond milk

1 fats-loose and sugar-loose chocolate instant pudding package deal deal

1 cup low-fat whipped cream

¼ teaspoon dried ginger

1 tablespoon almonds, overwhelmed (non-obligatory)

Directions:

Pour bloodless milk right right into a mixing bowl and, beating step by step with wire whisk, add the pudding combination and dried ginger. Keep whisking for 2 mins. Fold inside the cool whip topping.

Spoon into pudding cups, refrigerate for as a minimum three hours.

Garnish with almonds surely in advance than serve, if desired.

Nutrition: Calories: 302 - Fat: 25 g - Protein: 4 g - Carbs: 21 g - Fiber: 9 g - Sugar: 7 g

41. Asparagus and Arugula Salad

Preparation Time: 5 mins

Cooking Time: 10 minutes

Servings: 2

Ingredients:

½ bunch asparagus, trimmed

2 cups little one arugula

1 tablespoon balsamic vinegar

1 tablespoon greater-virgin olive oil

2 radishes, thinly sliced

2 tablespoons low-salt feta cheese, crumbled

A pinch sea salt

A pinch black pepper

Cooking spray

Directions:

Put the asparagus in your air fryer basket, grease with cooking spray, season with salt and pepper and prepare dinner at 360 °F for 10 mins.

In a bowl, stir the asparagus with the arugula, season with the vinegar, olive oil, salt and pepper and blend nicely.

Divide amongst plates and serve with feta sprinkled on pinnacle.

Nutrition: Calories: two hundred - Fat: nine g - Protein: 6 g - Carbs: 14 g - Fiber: 5 g - Sodium: 384 mg

forty two. Mushrooms and Cheese Spread

Preparation Time: five minutes

Cooking Time: 20 minutes

Servings: 2

Ingredients:

1 cup white mushrooms

¼ cup low-fats mozzarella, shredded

1 cup low-fats cream cheese

½ tablespoon parsley, finely chopped

½ garlic clove, minced

A pinch sea salt

A pinch black pepper

Cooking spray

Directions:

Put the mushrooms on your air fryer basket, grease with cooking spray, and prepare dinner dinner at 370 °F for 20 mins.

Place mushrooms and ultimate additives proper into a blender and pulse well, till gentle and spreadable.

Nutrition: Calories: 162 - Fat: 7 g - Protein: 7 g - Carbs: 8 g - Fiber: 2 g - Sodium: 326 mg

43. Zucchini Squash Mix

Preparation Time: 10 mins

Cooking Time: 35 minutes

Servings: four

Ingredients:

½ lb. Zucchini, sliced

1 medium yellow squash, halved, deseeded and chopped

½ onion, diced

1 tablespoon parsley, chopped

1 teaspoon thyme

1 tablespoon olive oil

A pinch sea salt

A pinch pepper

Directions:

Into a large bowl, add all factors and mix properly.

Transfer into the air fryer basket and prepare dinner at 4 hundred °F for 35 mins. Serve and experience.

Nutrition: Calories: seventy nine - Fat: five g - Protein: 2 g - Carbs: 6 g - Sugar: 2 g - Cholesterol: 0 mg

44. Tomatoes with Basil and Garlic

Preparation Time: 10 mins

Cooking Time: 12 minutes

Servings: 2

Ingredients:

1 cup cherry tomatoes, halved

½ bunch basil, chopped

1 ½ garlic cloves, minced

A drizzle olive oil

Sea salt and black pepper, to taste

Directions:

In a pan that suits your air fryer, combine tomatoes with garlic, salt, pepper, basil and oil, and mix till nicely combined.

Introduce in your air fryer and prepare dinner at 320 °F for 12 minutes. Divide among plates and characteristic a issue dish.

Nutrition: Calories: sixty two - Fat: 3 g - Protein: 2 g - Carbs: 4 g - Fiber: 1 g - Sodium: 15 mg

45. Chicken Alfredo

Preparation Time: 15 minutes

Cooking Time: sixteen minutes

Servings: four-6

Ingredients:

1 lb. Fowl breasts, skinless and boneless

½ lb. Button mushrooms, sliced

1 medium-sized onion, chopped

five oz. Mild Alfredo sauce

½ teaspoon dried thyme

Black pepper, to taste

Cooking spray

Directions:

Cut the hen breasts into 1 inch cubes.

Mix bird, onion, and mushrooms in a massive bowl. Season with pepper and dried thyme, and mix nicely.

Preheat your air fryer to 370 °F and grease basket with cooking spray.

Transfer chicken and greens to the air fryer and cook dinner for 12 minutes, stirring once in a while.

Stir in the Alfredo sauce. Cook for every other 4 minutes.

Nutrition: Calories: 289 - Fat: 12 g - Protein: thirteen g - Carbs: 19 g - Sodium: 493 mg

forty six. Perfect Crab Dip

Preparation Time: five minutes

Cooking Time: 7 minutes

Servings: 6

Ingredients:

1 ½ cup crab meat

2 tablespoons parsley, chopped

2 tablespoons sparkling lemon juice

2 tablespoons low-carb warmness sauce

½ cup green onion, sliced

1 cup low-fats cheese, grated

¼ cup low-fat mayonnaise

¼ teaspoon pepper

A pinch sea salt

Directions:

In a 6 inch dish, mixture collectively crab meat, heat sauce, onion, cheese, mayo, pepper, and salt.

Place dish in air fryer basket and prepare dinner dip at four hundred °F for 7 minutes.

Remove dish from air fryer.

Drizzle dip with lemon juice and garnish with parsley. Serve and enjoy.

Nutrition: Calories: 288 - Fat: 23 g - Protein: thirteen g - Carbs: 6 g - Sodium: 431 mg

47. Crab-Stuffed Mushrooms

Preparation Time: 10 minutes

Cooking Time: 8 minutes

Servings: 2

Ingredients:

4 oz... Mushrooms, cleaned and stems chopped

¼ teaspoon chili powder

¼ teaspoon onion powder

¼ cup low-fats mozzarella cheese, shredded

2 oz.. Crab meat, chopped

2 oz... Fat-loose cream cheese, softened

1 teaspoon garlic, minced

1 tablespoon inexperienced onion, finely chopped

¼ teaspoon pepper

Directions:

Preheat the air fryer to 370 °F. Line the air fryer basket with baking paper.

In a blending bowl, stir stems, chili powder, onion powder, pepper, mozzarella, crab meat, cream cheese, and garlic till well blended.

Stuff mushroom caps with bowl aggregate and region into the air fryer basket.

Cook for eight minutes.

Remove from the air fryer and top with green onion. Serve and revel in.

Nutrition: Calories: 139 - Fat: eight g - Protein: five g - Carbs: four g - Sodium: 228 mg

forty eight. Zucchini with Salmon Fillets

Preparation time: four mins

Cooking time: 10 mins

Servings: 2

Ingredients:

Canola oil – 2 tbsp.

Onion (chopped) – 1

Zucchini (chopped) – 1-

Salmon fillets – 1 lb.

Black beans – three cups

Tomatoes (diced) – 2

Salt and pepper to taste

Corn – ½ cup

Parsley to garnish

Directions:

Add oil into the air fryer pot.

Mix salmon fillets, onion, black beans, tomatoes, corn, zucchini and salt and pepper.

Cook at three hundred F for 10 mins.

When done, garnish with parsley and serve.

Nutrition: Kcal 90 5 | Sodium: 595mg | Protein: 200g | Carbs: 10g | Fat: 6g | Potassium: 439mg

40 9. Black Beans with Ham and Salmon

Preparation time: 4 minutes

Cooking time: 9 mins

Servings: 3

Ingredients:

Ham hock – 2 lb.

Salmon (chopped) – 1 lb.

Onion (chopped) – 1

Garlic cloves (minced) – 2

Black beans – 2 cups

Bay leaves – 2

Oregano powder – 2 tbsp.

Directions:

Add onion and bay leaves into the air fryer pot.

Mix ham hock, garlic, black beans and oregano powder.

Cook at three hundred F for 9 minutes.

When finished, serve and experience the meal!

Nutrition: Kcal ninety five I Sodium: 423mg I Protein: 200g I Carbs: 10g I Fat: 6g I Potassium: 722mg

50. Tender Soft Mexican Chicken Salad

Preparation Time: five minutes

Cooking Time: 0 minutes

Servings: 2

Ingredients:

2 tsps. Juice of jarred salsa

1 tsp. Taco seasoning

1 tbsp. Light mayonnaise

1 C. Canned chook, drained

Directions:

Add the tired hen to a bowl and take a fork, smash the chicken into small portions.

Add mayonnaise to the chicken and integrate well, mash the chook into the mayonnaise with a fork.

Add the salsa juice and taco seasoning to the fowl mix, hold mixing and mash the entirety well.

Serve and revel in!

Nutrition: Calories: 284 Fat: 4 g. Carbs: 16 g. Protein: 6 g. Sodium: 430 mg.

51. Honeydew & Kiwi Infused Water

Preparation Time: five mins + 1 hour chilling time

Cooking Time: 0 minutes

Servings: 2

Ingredients:

1 kiwi, peeled and sliced

2 cups honeydew melon, chopped

10 cups Water

Directions:

In a glass integrate the culmination.

Fill to the pinnacle with water.

Refrigerate for 1 hour earlier than serving.

Nutrition: Calories 12 Total Fat 0.Zero g Carbohydrate 4.Four g Protein zero.Zero g

fifty two. Sweet and Sour Lychee Infused Water

Preparation Time: five mins + 1 hour chilling time

Cooking Time: zero mins

Servings: 2

Ingredients:

1 cup lychees, peeled, seeded

1 tbsp. Ginger powder

10 cups water

three tablespoons lemon juice

Directions:

Combine all of your materials in a glass.

Refrigerate for 1 hour in advance than serving.

Nutrition: Calories 2 Total Fat 0.Zero g Carbohydrate 31g Protein zero.Zero g

fifty three. Kiwi and Kale Detox Water

Preparation Time: 5 minutes + 1 hour chilling time

Cooking Time: zero mins

Servings: 2

Ingredients:

four kiwis, sliced

five kale leaves

10 cups bloodless water

Directions:

Combine all of your elements in a glass.

Refrigerate for 1 hour earlier than serving.

Nutrition: Calories 1.7 Total Fat 0.0g Carbohydrate eight g Protein 17 g

fifty 4. Watermelon and Lemon Water

Preparation Time: 10 mins

Cooking Time: 0 minutes

Servings: 2

Ingredients:

3 cups watermelon, chunks, seeded

three tablespoons lemon juice

2-three mint leaves

1 pinch salt

10 cups water

Directions:

Combine all of your elements in a glass.

Refrigerate for 1 hour in advance than serving.

Nutrition: Calories one zero 5.1 Total Fat 1.4 g Carbohydrate 24.6 g Protein 2.1 g

fifty five. Mango & Ginger Infused Water

Preparation Time: five mins + 3 hours chilling time

Chapter 12: Snacks and Appetizers

sixty 5. Raspberry Gelatin Tea

Preparation Time: five mins

Cooking Time: 5 mins

Servings: 1

Ingredients:

½ cup frozen raspberries, chopped

¼ teaspoon stevia, or low-calorie sweetener

2 easy mint leaves, finely chopped

½ cup warm water

2 tablespoons low-calorie simple gelatin powder

Directions:

In a small saucepan, stir inside the raspberries over medium warmness for 2 minutes, upload stevia, and prepare dinner dinner for 1 minute. Remove from the warmth and set apart.

Pour the new water right into a mug. Stir within the gelatin powder and upload in the raspberries and mint, stirring constantly.

In a mixer, tool the mixture until foamy, pour right into a mug, allow cool and revel in right now.

Nutrition: Calories: 93 - Fat: zero g - Protein: nine g - Carbs: eight g - Fiber: 1 g - Sugar: 4 g - Sodium: fifty 4 mg

sixty six. Cinnamon Vanilla Coconut Milk

Preparation Time: 1 hour to loosen up

Cooking Time: 5 mins

Servings: 1

Ingredients:

½ cup mild unsweetened coconut milk

2 teaspoons vanilla extract

1 teaspoon stevia, or low-calorie sweetener

¼ teaspoon cinnamon

1 teaspoon lemon zest

2 mint leaves, finely chopped

1 tablespoon low-calorie easy gelatin powder

Directions:

In a small saucepan, heat the coconut milk for 1-2 mins. Sprinkle in the vanilla extract, mint and stevia and stir to dissolve.

Add the gelatin on the same time as stirring continuously to dissolve the gelatin clearly. Remove from the warm temperature.

In a mixer, switch the aggregate and blend for some seconds until frothy, and pour right into a small mug.

Let set inside the refrigerator for about 1 hour. Serve and experience.

Nutrition: Calories: 139 - Fat: 8 g - Protein: 5 g - Carbs: 6 g - Fiber: zero g - Sugar: four g - Sodium: 71 mg

67. Yogurt, Chocolate and Chia Pudding

Preparation Time: 8 hours to take a seat returned

Cooking Time: zero minutes

Servings: 2

Ingredients:

½ cup unsweetened almond milk

½ cup non-fats simple Greek yogurt

2 tablespoons chia seeds

1 teaspoon unsweetened cocoa powder

¼ teaspoon ground cinnamon

⅛ teaspoon vanilla extract

½ teaspoon stevia, or no-calorie sweetener

1 tablespoon vanilla whey protein (non-obligatory)

Directions:

In small bowl, integrate the almond milk, yogurt, chia seeds, cocoa powder, stevia, vanilla extract, cinnamon, and whey protein (if the use of).

Cover and let sit down in fridge in a single day, or at least four-five hours, stirring after 1 hour that has been located within the refrigerator.

Nutrition: Calories: 209 - Fat: 10 g - Protein: 16 g - Carbs: 21 g - Fiber: 9 g - Sugar: eight g - Sodium: 98 mg

sixty eight. Mocha and Coffee Protein Shake

Preparation time: five minutes

Cooking time: zero mins

Servings: 2

Ingredients:

½ cup low-fat milk

1 cup decaffeinated coffee, brewed and chilled ¼ cup vanilla protein powder

1 teaspoon unsweetened cocoa powder

½ teaspoon vanilla extract

four ice cubes

Directions

Combine the milk, espresso, protein powder, cocoa powder, vanilla, and ice in a blender. Blend on excessive pace until actually smooth.

Half of the shake want to be poured into a glass and loved.

Refrigerate the final 1/2 in an airtight jar for as a wonderful deal as every week, then reblend earlier than serving.

Nutrition: electricity: 90 5 fats: 2.0g protein: 10.0g carbs: 9.0g internet carbs: nine.0g fiber: 0g

sixty nine. Fruit and Green Protein Shake

Preparation time: five mins

Cooking time: zero mins

Servings: 2

Ingredients:

1½ cups water

½ medium Avocado

½ small Granny Smith apple

2 loose handfuls spinach

1 small handful glowing parsley

¼ avocado, peeled

Juice of one lemon

¼ cup unflavored protein powder

Directions:

In a blender, integrate the water, Avocado, apple, spinach, parsley, avocado, lemon juice, and protein powder. Blend on excessive till clean.

Pour half of of the shake into a pitcher, and experience.

Store the final 1/2 of in an airtight field in the fridge for as much as in step with week, and reblend previous to serving.

Nutrition: electricity: 133 fats: five.0g protein: 10.0g carbs: sixteen.0g net carbs: 12.0g fiber: four.0g

70. Chocolate and Raspberry Protein Shake

Preparation time: five mins

Cooking time: zero minutes

Servings: 1

Ingredients:

1 cup low-fats milk

¼ cup chocolate protein powder

2 teaspoons unsweetened cocoa powder

1 teaspoon vanilla extract

½ cup frozen raspberries

Directions:

Combine the milk, protein powder, cocoa powder, vanilla, and raspberries in a blender. Blend on immoderate pace until genuinely clean.

Half of the shake have to be poured into a glass and loved.

Refrigerate the remaining 1/2 of in an airtight jar for as much as every week, then reblend in advance than serving.

Nutrition: energy: 285 fat: 5.0g protein: 27.0g carbs: 33.0g internet carbs: 27.0g 71. Puréed Squash Soup

Preparation Time: 10 mins

Cooking Time: half-hour

Servings: 6-8

Ingredients:

three cups butternut squash, chopped

four cups low-sodium vegetable inventory

2 garlic cloves, chopped

1 tablespoon olive oil

1 ½ cup unsweetened coconut milk

¾ tablespoon curry powder

½ teaspoon dried onion flakes

1 teaspoon kosher salt

Directions:

Add butternut squash, oil, onion flakes, curry powder, inventory, garlic, and salt right into a saucepan and bring to boil over medium-excessive warmth.

Turn warmness to medium and simmer for 20 minutes.

Purée the soup using an immersion blender until clean.

Return soup to the saucepan, stir in coconut milk, and put together dinner for 2-three minutes. Serve and experience.

Nutrition: Calories: a hundred and forty four - Fat: eight g - Protein: 3 g - Carbs: 19 g - Fiber: 4 g - Sugar: 5 g

seventy . Homemade Chicken Broth

Preparation Time: 15 minutes

Cooking Time: 2 ½ hours

Servings: 3

Ingredients:

1 lb. Bone-in, pores and pores and skin on hen

2 celery stalks, extra or less chopped

2 carrots, peeled and form of chopped

2 onions, quartered

1 garlic clove, peeled

½ tablespoon dried sage

½ tablespoon dried rosemary

½ tablespoon dried thyme

2 bay leaves

4 cups water

⅓ teaspoon floor pepper

A pinch of sea salt, to flavor

Directions:

Add all substances, besides salt, to a large pot over medium-excessive warmth and bring to a boil.

Remove foam because it includes the ground after which lower the warm temperature.

Let put together dinner blanketed for approximately 2 hours, till the pork is so easy that it comes off the bone effects.

Strain the broth, collect it in a bowl, and add salt.

Let it cool to room temperature after which location it within the fridge in a single day.

Remove any extra fats to be able to have come to the surface, reheat the broth and serve.

Nutrition: Calories: sixty five - Fat: 1 g - Protein: 13 g - Carbs: 1 g - Sodium: 2 hundred mg

73. Homemade Beef Broth

Preparation Time: 15 minutes

Cooking Time: three hours

Servings: 3

Ingredients:

1 lb. Bone-in pork meat (shank bones, rib bones, knuckle bones, and so forth.)

2 celery stalks, greater or less chopped

2 carrots, peeled and extra or much less chopped

1 onion, quartered

1 small leek, greater or less chopped

1 garlic clove, peeled

2 bay leaves

1 teaspoon juniper berries

½ tablespoon dried sage

½ tablespoon dried rosemary

½ tablespoon entire peppercorns

four cups water

A pinch of sea salt, to taste

Directions:

Add all additives, except salt, to a large pot over medium-excessive warmth and convey to a boil.

Lower the warmth and let prepare dinner dinner dinner included for approximately 3 hours getting rid of the froth that rises to the floor.

Strain the broth, acquire it in a bowl, and upload salt.

Let it cool to room temperature after which vicinity it inside the refrigerator in a single day.

Remove any extra fat that allows you to have come to the floor, reheat the broth and serve.

Nutrition: Calories: eighty - Fat: three g - Protein: 10 g - Carbs: 3 g - Sodium: 205 mg

seventy four. Creamy Avocado Soup

Preparation Time: 10 mins

Cooking Time: zero minutes

Servings: 2

Ingredients:

2 avocados, peeled and pitted

2 tablespoons smooth lemon juice

¾ cup light cream cheese

¼ cup cilantro

Sea salt and pepper, to taste

Directions:

Add avocado, lemon juice and cilantro to a blender and blend till smooth.

Pour mixed mixture proper proper right into a bowl.

Add cream and stir nicely. Season with pepper and salt. Serve and revel in.

Nutrition: Calories: 102 - Fat: 9 g - Protein: 3 g - Carbs: 6 g - Fiber: 5 g - Sugar: 2 g

75. Almond Protein Shake

Preparation Time: five mins

Cooking Time: five mins

Servings: 1

Ingredients:

2 tbsp. Almonds

1 scoop chocolate protein powder

12 ounces.. Unsweetened almond milk

1 c. Ice

2 tbsp. Coconut flakes

Directions:

Add all substances into the blender and mix till easy and creamy.

Serve and revel in.

Nutrition: Calories 214 Fat 5 g Carbohydrates eight.Eight g Sugar 2.1 g Protein 14 g

seventy six. Almond Butter Shake

Preparation Time: five minutes

Cooking Time: five minutes

Servings: 1

Ingredients:

three tbsp. Almond butter

1 c. Unsweetened almond milk

half of c. Ice

6 drops liquid stevia

1 tbsp. Coconut oil

1 tbsp. Unsweetened cocoa powder

Directions:

Add all substances into the blender and mix till easy and creamy.

Serve and experience.

Nutrition: Calories 245 Fat five g Carbohydrates 8.Five g Sugar 1 g Protein 6 g

seventy seven. Chocó Blackberry Shake

Preparation Time: 5 minutes

Cooking Time: 5 mins

Servings: 1

Ingredients:

1/4 c. Blackberries

1 c. Unsweetened coconut milk

1/2 of c. Ice

2 tbsp. MCT oil

1/four tsp xanthan gum

drops liquid stevia

2 tbsp. Unsweetened cocoa powder

Directions:

Add all substances into the blender and mix until smooth and creamy.

www.ingramcontent.com/pod-product-compliance
Lightning Source LLC
Chambersburg PA
CBHW051726020426
42333CB00014B/1175